SIMPLE PRINCIPLES®
TO QUIT SMOKING

Alex A. Lluch

Author of Over 3 Million Books Sold!

WS Publishing Group
San Diego, California

SIMPLE PRINCIPLES®
TO QUIT SMOKING

By Alex A. Lluch

Published by WS Publishing Group
San Diego, California 92119
Copyright © 2009 by WS Publishing Group

Designed by WS Publishing Group:
David Defenbaugh

For Inquiries:
Logon to www.WSPublishingGroup.com
E-mail info@WSPublishingGroup.com

ISBN 13: 978-1-934386-39-2

Printed in China

TABLE OF CONTENTS

INTRODUCTION

In 1986, Patrick Reynolds—grandson of tobacco giant R.J. Reynolds—courageously walked away from the family business to advocate for a smoke-free America. Citing the deaths of his father and brother from smoking-related illnesses as inspiration for championing his cause, Reynolds testified before Congress, supporting an advertising ban on tobacco products. In 1987, he testified again, this time helping to get smoking banned on airplanes.

Reynolds now speaks to students at elementary, middle, and high schools, as well as at universities, to educate people about the dangers of smoking. His goal is to talk kids out of smoking and adults into quitting by both educating and inspiring them to believe that cigarettes are never the answer to life's problems. But considering that 45.3 million people in the United States continue to smoke, despite the valiant efforts of Patrick Reynolds and others like him, is it even possible to be talked out of smoking?

Patrick Reynolds thinks so, and so do we. Talking yourself into quitting is just one way in which *Simple Principles® to Quit Smoking* will aid you in your plan to become smoke-free. It's just one of the ways in which this book helps you devise a personal smoking-cessation program that is bound to work—because it is based on your habit, your lifestyle, and your needs.

What is this book about?

This book is about building up the courage to quit smoking. It addresses all the steps leading up to your Quit Day, a day you choose based on a variety of factors in your life. But this book takes you well beyond Quit Day, focusing on a lifetime of smoke-free maintenance. This is because we realize that quitting smoking is more than a decision, more than throwing away your cigarettes, and more than getting through the withdrawal period. Indeed, smoking cessation is a process, and a lifelong one.

Mark Twain once quipped, "Giving up smoking is the easiest thing in the world. I know because I've done it thousands of times." His tongue-in-cheek take on smoking gets to the heart of what so many people find when they go to quit smoking—that giving up cigarettes is extremely difficult! It requires planning, 100 percent commitment, and diligence if you really want to succeed. *Simple Principles® to Quit Smoking* takes much of the guesswork and trial-and-error out of this process. It guides you through each step of the quitting process, helping you build the tools you need to quit and stay smoke-free. This is not to say that you won't experience slipups, relapses, second-guesses, and starting over—you might, and this book accounts for that. It helps you get over setbacks, deal with slipups, and turn your mistakes into valuable lessons that, in the end, will keep you smoke-free. In fact, one of the best features of this book is its realistic approach to quitting.

This book includes tips that will tell you what to do if you are tempted to smoke at a funeral, what to say if invited to a smoke-filled happy hour, how to manage stress, what foods to avoid, and how you can expect your health to improve once you quit. There are suggestions for what to do if you do slip and have 1 or 2 cigarettes, or if you completely relapse and smoke an entire pack. And finally, what this book sets out to prove is that there is no one way to quit smoking. Each person who makes the decision to stop smoking has his or her own reasons that must be taken into consideration when a cessation plan is being developed.

Who should read this book?

Simple Principles® to Quit Smoking is for anyone who wants to put out their last cigarette and free themselves from the slavery of nicotine addiction. It is for anyone who wants to avoid the increased health risks that come from smoking. It is for women who want to become—or are currently—pregnant but are so addicted to smoking they cannot imagine giving it up. It is for people who want to significantly decrease their risk for having a fatal smoking-related heart attack and for men and women who want to be alive and healthy to watch their children, grandchildren, and even great grandchildren grow up. It is for middle-aged men and women who are tired of spending $35 a week on cigarettes, instead of putting that money into a retirement account. This book is also for everyone who loves someone who smokes and wants to help them quit. In short, this book is for anyone who is somehow affected by the laundry-list of woes that come with smoking cigarettes.

This book is for people who want to:

- Learn how to get a handle on their smoking habit
- Understand how they became addicted to nicotine
- Figure out how much money they spend on cigarettes
- Target times when they are most likely to smoke
- Imagine how it feels to be a non-smoker
- Believe in their ability to quit smoking
- Learn new ways of coping with insecurity
- Know what smoking does to the body
- Understand the emotional toll smoking takes
- Learn to be unafraid of change
- Overcome the fear of letting go of old habits
- Trust that they will be able to function without cigarettes
- Know what steps to take to prepare to quit
- Develop a plan for giving up cigarettes
- Quit smoking by tapering off
- Learn about nicotine replacement therapy
- Avoid situations that tempt them to smoke

- Develop the willpower to quit
- Learn how to cope with the withdrawal period
- Avoid gaining weight after quitting
- Learn how to deal with stress without smoking
- Get back on track after a slipup or relapse
- Learn how quickly their body rebounds after quitting
- Stay smoke-free for life

Even if you are already in the midst of another smoking cessation program, you can benefit from this book. If there is one thing you will definitely learn from the 200 simple principles that follow it is that the more support you have when quitting smoking, the better your chances for success!

Why should you read this book?

You should read this book because you are tired of being tethered to the destructive habit of smoking—and because you are ready to throw out your pack and with it, all of the bad behaviors that encourage you to smoke. By picking up this book, you are acknowledging that something has to change and that you are no longer happy with being a smoker.

In reading it, you admit that the time has come to give up cigarettes forever. And by revisiting the 200 well-researched and thoughtful tips contained within these pages, you commit to living out the rest of your days as a non-smoker. These are the reasons you should read this book.

In case you are still not sure if this book is for you, ask yourself:

- Am I tired of spending so much money on cigarettes?
- Would I like whiter teeth and fresher breath?
- Wouldn't it be nice to smell great again?
- Do I have a persistent cough or trouble breathing?
- Does it take me a long time to recover from a cold?
- Has my doctor told me to give up smoking?
- Am I tired of standing out in the cold by myself?
- Has a family member or friend asked me to quit?
- Am I willing to give up the last 10 years of my normal life expectancy?
- Do I want my kids to smoke?
- Do I want to decrease my risk of developing lung cancer or of having fatal heart attack?

- Will I ever want to bear children?
- Do I want to risk losing my infant to SIDS?
- Do I really think I am invincible against the damage caused by smoking?
- Am I ready to make a positive change for my health?
- Do I want to create a plan to quit smoking for good?

Reading this book is just one part of your journey to becoming a non-smoker. Think of it as a road map with well-marked signs for how to proceed. It can be read straight-through, or you can read the chapters out of order, when you need them most. This book is a tool for you to incorporate into your quit-smoking plan as you see fit. Consider reading this book as the start of your new, non-smoking life. As Henry David Thoreau wrote in his masterpiece, *Walden*, "How many a man has dated a new era in his life from the reading of a book." Let *Simple Principles® to Quit Smoking* mark a new era in your life—the era of a smoke-free, healthier, happier you.

Quitting smoking for good!

You may have become so deeply entrenched in your habit at

this point in your life that you may barely be able to recall the time before you started smoking. But there was a time. That time is what you will think back to as you create your plan to stop smoking and start living.

It is important to remember that all smokers were made, not born. You had to work at becoming addicted to cigarettes—and now you must work to break that addiction. To help you, this book acknowledges the difficulty of quitting smoking, while also highlighting that giving up cigarettes is not really a sacrifice—it is a gift you give to yourself and to those who care about you. Indeed, when you look at nicotine addiction objectively, it becomes abundantly clear that quitting will be one of the best decisions you will ever make.

Why is it so difficult to quit smoking?

There are many reasons for why quitting smoking is so difficult. All these reasons fit into one of two simple categories. One is that tobacco companies spend big bucks to make smoking seem appealing, the other is that nicotine is a highly addictive substance. The combination of these two elements makes for a habit that is walled in by your perception of smoking, in addition to a serious physical addiction. Breaking through that wall is both scary and challenging, but completely possible.

This book will teach you how to reprogram your brain to combat what tobacco advertising has taught you about smoking. This will take work because, according to the Federal Trade Commission, tobacco companies spend $13.11 billion— or more than $35 million daily—to promote their products. But once you have a grip on the elements that make up your habit, you can chisel away at your beliefs about smoking. For example, if you smoke to unwind after work, you will be interested to know that nicotine is a stimulant that actually exacerbates irritability and prevents sleep. Knowing this is the first step to arming your brain against images that show a woman lounging on a beach, relaxing with a cigarette.

Your next step is to deal with your physical addiction. This part can either be easier or more difficult than the social aspect, depending on how much you smoke. According to the American Lung Association it only takes 7 seconds for nicotine to reach your brain when you inhale. If you smoke a pack a day for 20 years that means you have inhaled nicotine over a million times! Since your tolerance for the drug increases over time you tend to smoke more and become more addicted. Breaking this cycle is not easy to do, but the good news is that you are reading this book, which will equip you to deal with both the physical and mental components of quitting smoking.

What do you have to gain by quitting smoking?

In a word: everything. When you give up cigarettes you extend the length and quality of your life by drastically reducing your risk of developing dozens of smoking-related illnesses, many of which are fatal. In addition, you enrich the relationships you have with family and friends by showing them you care about yourself—and them—enough to make the effort to quit. Also, when you stop smoking you start caring more about other areas of your life that need improvement, such as your diet, mental health, and finances. Truly, the effort to quit smoking results in an overhaul that leaves every aspect of your life improved.

What do you need to know in order to quit for good?

The goal of staying quit is best envisioned as a bright and shiny star that you always follow but never quite reach. In other words, you must never feel as though you have completely achieved your goal or that you are "done," because becoming an ex-smoker is a lifelong process. It is an effort that becomes much easier as the years pass, but, like people who were once alcoholics or drug addicts, you must always consider yourself as having escaped your addiction to nicotine, but wary of conditions that may cause you to relapse.

Indeed, hold the goal of staying quit up as a beacon that guides you through the decisions you make for the rest of your life. Don't worry—it's not as hard as it sounds. By the time you do all the work to stop smoking, your mind-set will be that of a non-smoker.

Maximizing the Benefits of this Book

You will use this book to learn why you smoke, when you smoke, the reasons you smoke, and how much you spend on smoking. It is only after analyzing your habit that you can figure out how to stop. *Simple Principles® to Quit Smoking* will guide you step by step through the quitting process, an extremely challenging time. Let this book be your guide, your partner, your confidante. Then, after you have made it through the quitting process, let this book help you stay smoke-free for life. After you have successfully become an ex-smoker, let this book open the door to other lifestyle changes.

Always keep this book handy and read it often. Carry it in place of your cigarettes. Keep it in your purse or briefcase. Put it in the glove compartment of your car. Stick it in the top drawer of your desk in your office. Lay it on your nightstand before bed. This book is written to be read over and over again. Read it often to get ideas for how to deal with temptation and for on-the-go inspiration when you need a little boost. Most of all, incorporate the well-researched methods and more than 200 pieces of advice into your smoking-cessation program to help you learn to quit smoking for good.

GETTING A HANDLE ON YOUR HABIT

One of reasons quitting smoking is so difficult is because for many people, smoking is not just an activity: it is a habit. By definition, a habit is routine behavior done without thought. When thought is absent from behavior, it becomes automatic and thus difficult to get a true handle on. As billionaire Warren Buffet said, "Bad habits are like chains that are too light to feel until they are too heavy to carry."

Start to think about smoking as the chain whose weight you have been unaware of up until this point. Interestingly, the first phase of quitting smoking has nothing to do with quitting at all; instead, your job at this point is to understand, even analyze, your habit. Think of your task in the following way: How are you supposed to make a plan for quitting smoking when you have no idea what you are up against? In other words, without knowing why, when, or how many cigarettes you go through in a day, you cannot possibly become aware of how severe your habit actually is. And in the same way you probably wouldn't take on a project that was unclear or a job that you didn't know how to do, you must not attempt to quit smoking before you understand the extent of your habit.

A mistake many smokers make when they decide to quit is to skip the important, initial step of quantifying their habit. This often leads to relapses or giving up on quitting all together, because the smoker realizes his smoking habit is more entrenched than he ever dreamed. For most smokers, smoking has become a way of life, a behavior pattern that is not easily cast off. To wrap your mind around how entwined smoking is with the rest of your life, you must first become mindful of when, why, and how much you smoke.

Getting a handle on your smoking habit arms you with the knowledge required to make a sound plan for quitting. You will need to learn what makes you want to smoke and come face to face with how many cigarettes you actually smoke each day. These and the other principles in this chapter will help you get a critical handle on your habit.

Principle #1

Look before you smoke.

————— ❋ —————

One way to get a handle on your habit is to keep close track of your cigarette consumption. Do this by looking at how many are left in the pack each time you have a smoke. Becoming aware of how many cigarettes you are running through helps you avoid smoking absentmindedly. Counting your cigarettes prevents you from plowing through your pack and makes you aware of how large your smoking habit actually is. Be honest with yourself because this important step leads to accountability—a necessary component of quitting. As author Mildred Newman once advised, "We are accountable only to ourselves for what happens to us in our lives." Begin holding yourself accountable by keeping track of how many cigarettes you smoke every day.

PRINCIPLE #2

Figure out your smoking schedule.

———————— ✳ ————————

Many of us have a daily routine that is so automatic, it requires little to no thought to perform. This is especially true of smokers. The act of putting match to cigarette is so routine that you may have, once or twice, found yourself trying to light an already-lit cigarette. To truly assess the extent of your smoking habit, this mindlessness must be turned into mindfulness. One way to train your brain to be "on" when you smoke is to look at your watch each time you have a cigarette. Do you tend to smoke more in the morning? Late at night? Evenly throughout the day? Do you smoke more when it is rainy or sunny outside? Eventually, you will notice that you have a schedule, which will become a valuable tool when you are ready to devise a plan to quit.

Principle #3

Put yourself on the clock when you smoke.

❉

People are often astounded to discover how many hours they actually spend smoking. According to Marshall Brain, author of *The Teenager's Guide to the Real World*, a person with a 2-pack-a-day habit smokes 600,000 cigarettes in his lifetime. Since it takes 3 to 5 minutes to smoke just 1 cigarette, that person is spending 30,000 to 50,000 hours—a total of 3 to 5 years—smoking over the course of his lifetime! If you smoke 1 pack a day, 1.5 to 2.5 years of your life will spent on your smoking habit. Start counting how much of your life you spend smoking by calculating how many cigarettes you have a day—then imagine how those years might be better spent.

Principle #4

Start a smoking journal.

---- ✳ ----

Quitting smoking and losing weight are two of the most overwhelming, impossible-seeming tasks, and both require a major overhaul of a person's lifestyle. It is not surprising then that there are weight-loss techniques that can also be applied to quitting smoking. One crossover example is to create a smoking journal. Studies show that when dieters track connections between their mood and food consumption, they have more success in breaking bad eating habits. Do the same for your smoking habit. Dedicate a notebook to writing down what you were doing and how you felt before and after each cigarette. Keep track of what made you want that cigarette. Like a food diary, your smoking journal will reveal a pattern of triggers that can be avoided once you are ready to quit.

Principle #5

Pay attention to what is in your other hand.

❋

Without thinking, many people pair their cigarettes with another activity, such as driving, playing music, and drinking coffee or alcohol. Others smoke while walking or talking on the phone. When smoking is absentmindedly paired with another activity, it becomes even more routine. By paying attention to what is in your other hand, you can get clued in to how you enhance your smoking experience by coupling it with other activities. Once you understand these triggering activities, you can figure out what to avoid when you feel the urge to smoke. Start paying attention to what is in one hand when you smoke, because it is likely causing you to hold a cigarette in the other.

Principle #6

Note how you feel while smoking.

————————————— ❋ —————————————

When you get the urge for a cigarette, take note of how you feel. Are you bored? Are you anxious, or having trouble concentrating? Did you just end an upsetting phone call? Have you been drinking? Next, pay attention to how you feel after you light up. Are you still anxious? Still bored? Still worried or upset? If so, you are not alone. According to Allen Carr, author of *The Easy Way to Stop Smoking*, smoking does not alleviate these feelings, but rather intensifies them through a preoccupation with thinking that a cigarette is the antidote to them. Worse, when a person still experiences these feelings after smoking, they light another cigarette, believing *this* is the one that will change how they feel. Realizing what your expectations of relief are helps get a handle on your habit.

PRINCIPLE #7

Admit how you really feel after a cigarette.

———————— ✳ ————————

Most people who have tried to quit are familiar with the pangs of regret that seep in after a night that started with, "I'll just have a puff," and ended with buying a fresh pack of cigarettes. Indeed, smoking is rarely confined to "just one" and usually causes both regret and the guilty desire for another cigarette, which inevitably circles back to regret. This cycle results in smoking expectations that are always met with disappointment and guilt. Admitting this to be true is an important step in assessing what you actually get out of your smoking habit. Noticing that you are participating in a cycle of addiction helps you see how destructive your smoking habit truly is.

PRINCIPLE #8

Track the expense of your habit by keeping receipts.

— ❋ —

To assess how much you spend on cigarettes, collect receipts for every pack purchased in the course of a month. Keep them in a safe place and make sure to get a receipt every time you buy a pack. You will be surprised by how much your habit costs. At $4.50 per pack, the average smoker spends around $1,638 per year on cigarettes! This money could be better spent on retirement, according to Hilary Smith, of MSN.com Money. Smith reports that quitting at age 40 and investing money formerly used for cigarettes into an investment account that earns 9 percent interest would add up to about $250,000 by the time you are 70! Even those who aren't motivated by money must take notice of this impressive statistic.

Principle #9

Map out where you smoke.

--- ❋ ---

The Buddha once said, "Just as a picture is drawn by an artist, surroundings are created by the activities of the mind." Consider how your smoking habit influences your surroundings. Are there places in which you smoke more than others? Do your surroundings suffer as a result of your habit? Take a moment to picture yourself in the places you most often smoke, and then consider how it makes you feel. For example, taking smoke breaks next to a dumpster in an alley may cause you to feel depressed, while smoking in your kitchen may be your way of hiding from your family. Becoming aware of where you smoke and the impact these places have on you will be a big piece of your quitting program, as environment plays a large role in a smoking habit.

PRINCIPLE #10

Imagine a conversation with your smoking buddies—without cigarettes.

———————————— ✳ ————————————

The social component of smoking is one of the most difficult parts of the habit to overcome. After all, smokers bond over their habit. This mini-community is attractive because it offers an immediate connection with a built-in ice-breaker: "Do you have a light?" However, keeping these folks in your life is likely to hinder your quitting efforts. In fact, a Brown University Medical School study found that adolescents who surrounded themselves with friends who smoked were 10 times more likely to become regular smokers. Evaluate whether your smoking relationships extend beyond the ashtray. If not, it may be time to extinguish them.

Principle #11

Be honest about your calculations.

— ❋ —

American entertainer Pearl Bailey once said, "The first and worst of all frauds is to cheat one's self. All sin is easy after that." Bailey's words ring true for a variety of life's challenges, and especially that of quitting smoking. If you are going to accurately assess your smoking habit, you must be 100 percent honest about what you discover. If you lie to yourself about your habit, it becomes easier to sneak cigarettes here and there. In this way, you cheat yourself out of quitting. Of course, it may be difficult to come face-to-face with the fact that you spend $150 a month on cigarettes, or that you actually smoke a pack-and-a-half a day, not a pack as you thought. But using true stats is the only way to get your arms around the whole problem and be able to dismantle it bit by bit.

Principle #12

Own up to behaviors
that help you cover up your habit.

Smokers engage in some interesting behaviors to sneak their habit into their lives. For example, a woman who does not want cigarettes to discolor her fingers might wear a rubber dish glove while she smokes. A businessman may wear an overcoat in hot weather to prevent the smell of smoke from clinging to his clothes. These behaviors create distance between the smoker and the unpleasantness associated with his habit. Identify any strange behaviors you engage in that allow you to distance yourself from the reality of your habit. Identifying these sneaky tricks forces you to confront the fact that you are a smoker and that you do need to quit.

Principle #13

Categorize your habit.

—— ✳ ——

Once you have collected information on your habit, categorize yourself as a light, medium, or heavy smoker. Light smokers are those who have just a couple of cigarettes a day—perhaps one after lunch and one before bed. A heavy smoker is someone who smokes a pack or more a day, and a moderate smoker is somewhere in between. When categorizing your habit, it is important to be honest! Admitting that you are a heavy smoker when you thought you smoked only moderately can be painful, but owning up to it is crucial to assessing your habit and determining how difficult it will be to quit. Categorizing your level of addiction will drive your cessation plan, so be brutally honest with yourself at this stage of the game.

Principle #14

Don't judge, just notice.

———————————— ❈ ————————————

Getting a handle on your smoking habit is an act of self-education that is intended to prepare you to quit. As such, it is important to avoid passing judgment on your personal smoking statistics as you assess your habit. Never think, "I'm such a loser! I can't believe I smoked 25 cigarettes today!" Doing so will cause you to feel like a failure before you even begin your cessation program. Instead, become a neutral observer of the facts so that you can create a plan that optimizes your chances for successfully quitting. If you are tempted to judge yourself, think instead of what philosopher and essayist George Santayana meant when he said: "The aim of education is the condition of suspended judgment on everything."

Imagining Yourself
as a Non-Smoker

Imagination inspires great works of art, literature, and music. It also creates powerful mental pictures when you read or listen. Imagination is so potent, in fact, that self-help experts such as Tony Robbins, Louise L. Hay, and Wayne Dyer have built entire empires on its power to change people's lives. Harnessing the power of your imagination is an important part of quitting smoking. The sheer act of imagining the benefits of being a non-smoker is enough to lay the groundwork for this change. As poet Samuel Taylor Coleridge once wrote, "Imagination is the living power and prime agent of all human perception."

The imagination is strong enough to help your mind accept the absence of cigarettes in your life. But training your mind to revise years of programmed associations with quitting smoking will take work. Previously, you have probably only imagined life as a non-smoker as being frustrating and miserable. Perhaps you have envisioned yourself overcome with craving and desire, tearing your hair out. Clearly, this sort of image does not cast quitting in a positive light! To reframe your image of yourself as a non-smoker, use positive associations that make you feel calm and capable. For example, when you picture a day without cigarettes, instead of imagining that you will feel anxious, deprived, and miserable, imagine yourself as active, satisfied, healthy, and confident.

An effective way to train your imagination is to focus on a time before you smoked. Imagine yourself at 10 or 12 years old—as a young, strong, and healthy non-smoker. Imagine that you never started smoking. Transport yourself to a time when quitting was not an issue, because there was nothing to give up. Focusing on this time is important for imagining your identity as a non-smoker, because it contains all the tools and good feelings you need to get back to a place in which you have no relationship with cigarettes. Indeed, there is no better way to imagine yourself as a non-smoker than by revisiting the time before you picked up your first cigarette. This idea and the following simple principles will help you in that endeavor.

Principle #15

Picture an additional $30 a week in your wallet.

❋

After figuring out how much you spend weekly on cigarettes, picture spending that money on other things. The average smoker spends about $126 a month on cigarettes, so use that as a starting point. What better ways might you envision spending this chunk of change? At today's prices, an extra $126 would buy you 4 or 5 concert tickets; a nice dinner in a fancy restaurant; a new dress; a couple weeks' worth of groceries; 120 songs from iTunes; 4 tanks of gas; a 90-minute massage; a plane ticket to a nearby city; a night in a bed and breakfast; or 12 copies of this book! Add up the financial benefits of quitting smoking and then imagine yourself enjoying them.

Principle #16

Imagine having an additional $97,000 to retire with.

❋

According to the U.S. Department of Labor, a person needs 70 percent of their pre-retirement income to maintain their standard of living in retirement. But in these tough economic times, many people are worrying if they have enough money saved. Yet as a smoker, you are sitting on a gold mine! By one estimate, a pack-a-day smoker who quits when they are 35 years old will have, if they put their cigarette money into a retirement account that earns 7 percent interest, an additional $97,000 by age 70. As you can see, it really does pay to be a non-smoker.

Principle #17

Imagine taking a deep breath in the morning—without coughing.

———— ✳ ————

Every smoker knows the morning routine of hacking up phlegm for 10 minutes before being able to take "a good breath." Some have worse coughs than others, but nearly all smokers have ways of dealing with it—hot showers, menthol chest rubs, an endless supply of tissues. Smokers cough because smoke causes airways to swell, making it difficult to clear the lungs. Imagine waking up with clear lungs and being able to take a phlegm-free breath. No matter how heavy a smoker you are, this vision is 100 percent possible—the U.S. Institutes of Health National Institute on Aging say that within just a few months of quitting, breathing becomes noticeably easier.

Principle #18

Watch the instant replay of you running across the finish line.

❊

Smokers often avoid physical challenges because smoking limits their ability to exercise. Indeed, smoke minimizes oxygen absorption throughout the body, causing dizziness, lethargy, and nausea. In addition, the need to have a cigarette every few hours discourages endeavors such as hiking or running long distances. To get motivated to quit, picture yourself as a non-smoker who is physically able to run a marathon. Imagine each detail, including the shoes and outfit—even pick a number to pin on your shirt. Finally, see yourself crossing the finish line. Watch spectators clap and roar for you, because you did it—you ran your first marathon as non-smoker!

Principle #19

Look at photos of yourself that were taken before you started smoking.

———————————— ✳ ————————————

Looking at photographs taken before you began smoking—even if you started very young—is a great way to see yourself as a non-smoker. These photos will remind you of what life was like B.C. (before cigarettes!). Think back: Who were you before cigarettes? What did you like to do? How did you fill your time? Chances are you were healthier, more active, and better looking. You probably smiled more because your teeth were not yellowed, and you did not suffer from chronic bad breath. You probably had more money and were definitely free from addiction. Stare at these photos often, feel how it was to be this person, and know that you will be that person again.

Principle #20

Imagine having the power to say no.

———————— ✳ ————————

Right now it may seem impossible to imagine saying no to a cigarette. In fact, turning down a cigarette may go against every fiber of your being. But you will get there eventually, and you should start by practicing how powerful it feels to say no to smoking. Self-help experts agree that establishing boundaries is often the most important step of self-empowerment. Indeed, self-empowerment will be the cornerstone of your cessation program. So, picture yourself as a non-smoker who is above the urge to smoke—practice not even being tempted by the offer. Do this by imagining someone has offered you a cigarette. Walk by this person and casually say, "No thanks. I don't smoke." Before you know it, you will be addicted not to cigarettes, but to the power of saying no.

PRINCIPLE #21

Look in the mirror and say,
"I am a non-smoker."

— ✳ —

Mirror, mirror on the wall, who's that non-smoker standing tall? It's you! Or it will be, and one day soon. Start practicing for that day now by imagining yourself as a non-smoker. Each moment you spend envisioning yourself as a non-smoking person brings you closer to that reality. Louise L. Hay, a visualization and self-empowerment expert, has commented on the power of seeing yourself as something you want to become. "You will see the little miracles occur in your life," she writes. "The things you are ready to eliminate will go of their own accord… You will get bonuses you never imagined!" Start looking at yourself as a non-smoker, and pretty soon you will be one.

Principle #22

Imagine running beside your grandchildren.

---- ❊ ----

An odd thing about smokers is how many of them allow themselves to accept the reality that they will likely die from a smoking-related illness. Some even use this likelihood to justify continuing their habit! You or a smoker you know might have joked, "If smoking doesn't kill me, something else will, so why should I quit now?" These statements are counterproductive. They encourage feelings of powerlessness instead of control. Change this mind-set by imagining yourself running with your grandchildren in a large field. Note the vivid colors that surround you; smell the fresh-cut grass. Feel how easy it is to breathe while running after your loved ones.

Principle #23

Visualize your lungs as pink and healthy.

———————————— ❊ ————————————

It only takes a few minutes of searching the Internet to find horrific pictures of lungs blackened and damaged from years of smoking. Though this shocking brand of image therapy has its place, focusing on healing is more productive to your psyche right now. So, sit in a quiet room and imagine that your lungs are a bright, burning red. Imagine that at the bottom of your lungs sits a cool, blue, healing liquid. Take deep breaths, and as you exhale imagine the liquid rising up, coating your lungs with cool relief, healing any wounds. The damage you've done to your lungs can be reversed, and it starts by imagining it.

PRINCIPLE #24

Sketch what you imagine
a non-smoker's life to be like.

Though not everyone is an artist, all of us are able to express some version of our ideas on paper. Scrawl out a few images of what you think a non-smoker's life might look like. You might draw a stick figure playing baseball with his son. Or, you might sketch a woman with pretty white teeth, clean clothes, driving somewhere in a brand new, smoke-free car. One study that had smokers do this exercise found the majority drew an activity they are currently unable to participate in but would do if they were a non-smoker. Adopting the life of a non-smoker seems more possible if you surround yourself with these kinds of images—so hang them all over the house!

PRINCIPLE #25

Write the story of the rest of your smoke-free life.

—— ✳ ——

Though it is not possible to know exactly how the rest of your life will turn out, writing your vision of how you want it to be is an important tool for change. The writer Franz Kafka once said, "A book must be the axe for the frozen sea inside us." Ponder these words as you work to create a story that breaks up your attachment to your identity as a smoker. As Kafka knew, writing causes one to engage their imagination and intellect to make a unique telling out of a common story. So, start writing. Your story of life as a non-smoker will be unique, compelling, and most importantly, will function as a guide for your life beyond cigarettes.

Principle #26

See yourself as an infant.

---- ✳ ----

It may sound strange to imagine yourself as an infant, but this is a common visualization exercise for people fighting addictions. Its usefulness makes sense when you consider the ways in which one must care for an infant. Certainly, you would not give an infant poisons such as tar and nicotine! Instead, see yourself as a baby with new lungs, hands, eyes— new everything, in fact. Over time, this image will create a desire to care for your body as if it was new and undamaged. Seeing yourself as priceless and vulnerable as a newborn baby is an important piece of your cessation program. It may help to carry a photograph of you as a baby to really zero in on this exercise.

Building the Confidence to Quit

It seems obvious that in order to successfully quit smoking, you must believe that you can do it. Yet most smokers start their cessation programs expecting to fail. And though statistically it may take smokers between 5 and 7 attempts to quit, studies repeatedly show that changing a pessimistic mind-set to an optimistic one dramatically increases your self-confidence—and therefore, your chances for long-term success. As the Reverend Jesse Jackson once said, "If my mind can conceive it, and my heart can believe it, I know I can achieve it." This sentiment is especially true about smoking.

Interestingly, countless studies show that boosting your confidence benefits all areas of your life, not just your attempt to quit smoking. *The Importance of Self-Confidence in Performance*, a study by Stephanie L. Stolz for Missouri Western State University, looked at the connection between self-confidence and athletic performance. Stolz found that athletes with higher self-confidence consistently outperformed those with lesser confidence in their abilities.

Of course, building up confidence in your ability to quit smoking will take time and effort. And the longer you have been smoking, the more challenging it is to believe you can live a smoke-free life. Therefore, gauging your confidence level before you start your cessation program is a useful first step. Ask yourself: When I think about quitting smoking, do I immediately feel defeated? Am I tempted to forget the whole thing? Do I often think, "I will never be a non-smoker"? If you answered yes to any of these questions, you have a confidence problem.

The principles in this chapter will help you tear down these destructive thoughts and replace them with confidence-building affirmations. One example of an empowering affirmation is to repeat, "I am stronger than my nicotine addiction." Focusing on such positive thoughts builds up your confidence to quit—which is exactly what you need right now. Use this and the following principles to guide you to a place of confidence in your ability to quit smoking for good.

Principle #27

Be willing to take care of yourself.

———————— ❊ ————————

It is surprising how many people don't take care of themselves. They put the needs of others ahead of their own until there is no time or energy left for self-care. Should a doctor advise this person to cut back on work, get more sleep, exercise, or quit smoking, he is often met with the stubborn retort of, "I don't have time." In order to quit smoking, you are going to have to make time. Treat your effort to quit smoking as a project that needs your attention. Start thinking of your health as a job that is as critical as the one that sends you a paycheck. Carving out space for self-care sends a clear message to yourself and to those around you that *you* matter. When you truly believe this, you will have achieved the courage to quit smoking.

Principle #28

Make sure your basic needs are met.

---------- ❈ ----------

In our busy culture, basic needs, such as proper nutrition, exercise, and sleep often take a backseat to work, family, and other pressing priorities. But 1960s psychologist Abraham Maslow discovered that is impossible to meet higher-level needs without addressing these basic needs first. It makes sense that a person who regularly forgoes his basic needs feels rundown and depressed. Over time, this negative routine depletes self-esteem. Make sure you are meeting your basic needs, such as eating regular, healthy meals; exercising 3 to 5 times a week; and getting enough rest. Satisfying your most basic needs breeds the self-confidence needed to quit smoking.

PRINCIPLE #29

Be a good parent to your inner child.

———————————— ❊ ————————————

There is an inner child within each of us. According to therapist Penny Parks, author of *Rescuing the Inner Child*, this inner child must be "re-parented" by our adult selves. Re-parenting your inner child is an opportunity to give positive messages to your inner self, such as, "It's not your fault" or, "You did your best." Such messages help release bottled-up guilt, anger, and shame. Letting go of these destructive feelings makes room for positive affirmations, which, in turn, boosts self-esteem. Additionally, all this work on the inner child sets you free from old issues that tether you to destructive habits like smoking, and paves the way to quitting for good.

Principle #30

Recognize you are in a codependent relationship.

✳

A codependent relationship is an unhealthy attachment to a person or substance that, over time, whittles away at your pride and self-esteem. These attachments tear you down rather than build you up. In fact, those in codependent relationships constantly feel forced to justify their attachments to anyone who will listen—including themselves. Sound familiar? It should, because smokers always have a million reasons for why they can't quit. What are some of yours? Instead of trotting out the same tired excuses, recognize you are in a codependent relationship with cigarettes. Then, admit it is time to break up with your smoking addiction.

PRINCIPLE #31

Build an invisible shield.

The inability to set boundaries is a classic symptom of a person who has low self-esteem. But as lifestyle makeover expert Cheryl Richardson has discussed, setting personal boundaries is like having an "invisible shield" that protects you from undeserved psychological harm. This shield also helps boost your sense of power. Practice setting boundaries in firm and simple language, such as, "I will not attend a party where I will be tempted to smoke." Build your invisible shield out of these promises. The invisible shield is a great tool for ratcheting up your self-confidence as you prepare to do battle with your smoking habit.

Principle #32

Prepare to cut out negative influences.

❋

An estimated 1.3 billion people worldwide smoke in spite of well-known health risks, rising cigarette costs, and negative public image. Make that one person less by vowing to cut smoking out of your life. To do this, you will need to cut out the negative influences that encourage or make it easier for you to smoke. Make a list of the people who negatively influence you. Identify anyone who chips away at your self-esteem. Examples include the friend who tells you are selling out because you want to quit smoking, or the coworker who bets that you will fail. Once your list is complete, ruminate on why these people made it to paper and then come up with a plan to limit your contact with them.

Principle #33

Stop hiding behind a pack of cigarettes.

——————— ✳ ———————

One reason people smoke is because they are uncomfortable in social situations. Indeed, standing in a group of people without smoking is torture for a person who subconsciously smokes to feel interesting or busy. It also explains why so many smokers start young, when they lack the social confidence gained later in life. To quit smoking, you must become comfortable enough to come out from behind your cigarettes. Instead of going outside for a smoke next time you are at a gathering, engage with your companions. Do as spiritual teacher and author Eileen Caddy advised: "Get into action and live this full and glorious life. Now. You have to do it." Better to spark an interesting conversation than a cigarette.

Principle #34

Find new ways to cope
with disappointment.

———————————— ✳ ————————————

People who suffer from low self-esteem have difficulty putting even the smallest disappointments into perspective. In fact, simple letdowns become four-alarm emotional emergencies that send the smoker straight to lighting a cigarette. Therefore, inventing new methods of coping is essential to your cessation program—and also to your confidence level. Indeed, people who are unable to deal with disappointment tend to spiral into self-doubt and pity, which leads to destructive behaviors. Next time you are tempted to pity yourself, reflect on what went wrong and come up with a plan for the future, rather than reaching for yet another cigarette.

Principle #35

Accept that you may not be the life of the party.

———————— ✳ ————————

People who feel socially awkward sometimes do everything in excess to become the life of the party. This gregarious persona is propped up by eating and drinking too much, smoking too much, and talking too much. In fact, this person may feel like it is impossible for them to be comfortable if something isn't going in or coming out of their mouth. This behavior is rooted in insecurity and can be controlled by building up self-esteem. When you feel the urge to turn the spotlight on yourself by having another cigarette, take 5 deep breaths and walk around the room. After awhile, it will feel more natural to engage with people on a less manic level.

Principle #36

At parties, use your hands to help serve and clean up.

———————— ✳ ————————

Those who suffer from social phobia and insecurity find it difficult to be in a group of people without smoking. Often they have no idea what to do with their hands. Clinical hypnotherapist Dr. Randy Gilchrist, author of *The Non-Smoker's Edge*, suggests that smokers need to find other ways of busying their hands for at least the first 6 months after quitting to reduce the likelihood of relapse. One suggestion is to occupy your hands by helping your host run the party. The constant action of refreshing drinks, serving food, and throwing out trash will keep your hands busy and cigarette-free all night.

PRINCIPLE #37

Cultivate assertiveness.

—— ❈ ——

Author Joan Didion once said, "To free us from the expectations of others, to give us back to ourselves—there lies the great, singular power of self-respect." In order to successfully transform from a smoker into a non-smoker, you must have self-respect. Therefore, you must become assertive—assertiveness is the lynchpin of self-confidence. Practice making assertive statements that do not include apologies or explanations. For example, say, "I am not interested in smoking right now." Resist the urge to hem, haw, explain, or backpedal. If you are unable to clearly let others know what you want, need, or reject, you will feel powerless and frustrated and will be more likely to give in to the pressure to have a cigarette.

PRINCIPLE #38

Express your feelings more often.

✳

An old saying goes, "Anger is only one letter short of the word danger." Indeed, there are few more destructive emotions than anger. Over time, anger depletes a person's feelings of self-worth, prohibiting progress and change. In order to prevent this negative spiral from impacting your effort to quit smoking, practice using "I" statements to communicate your feelings. An example might be, "I was disappointed that you did not attend my birthday party." This simple phrase claims your right to disappointment without assaulting the other person with unnecessary drama. Regularly exercising your right to such expression will prevent you from accumulating a backlog of anger, which will inevitably tempt you to smoke.

Principle #39

Use positive affirmations to quit procrastinating.

———————— ✳ ————————

Metaphysical author Louise L. Hay teaches that negative thought patterns lead to procrastination. This rings true when you think of how many attempts to quit never got off the ground because you told yourself, "I can't do this!" Hay proposes that instead of tearing yourself down with what you can't do, tell yourself what you can do. This facilitates change rather than making you feel like a failure. As Hay has eloquently put it, "Procrastination is one way to keep us from getting to where we say we want to go." Tell yourself you *can* quit smoking, and do so often. Building confidence in your ability to quit will get you there faster than you ever thought possible.

UNDERSTANDING THE HEALTH RISKS OF SMOKING

Smoking accounts for an estimated 438,000 of the 2.4 million annual deaths in the United States. According to the Surgeon General, smoking kills more people each year than HIV, illegal drugs, alcohol, motor vehicle accidents, suicides, and murders—*combined*. In addition to dying prematurely, smokers are at higher risk for stroke, all types of cancer, respiratory problems, and coronary heart disease, among several other chronic conditions.

The Surgeon General, American Heart Association, American Lung Association, American Cancer Society, and the Centers for Disease Control all agree that cigarette smoking is the single most preventable cause of death in the United States. And yet 20.8 percent—or 45.3 million—American adults continue to smoke cigarettes. Worse, 4,000 kids between ages 12 and 17 start smoking every day. Clearly, there is a disconnect between knowing the dangers of smoking and truly understanding how they affect individual smokers.

In order to successfully quit smoking, you must personalize the risk at which you put yourself every time you light a cigarette. Admittedly, it is difficult to apply impersonal statistics to your own life. Reading that 10 million people in the United States have been diagnosed with chronic obstructive pulmonary disease (COPD) may not impact you until you really imagine it affecting you. COPD prevents air from freely flowing through airways and results in chronic bronchitis and/or emphysema. Over time, damaged airways continue to obstruct airflow, eventually leading to suffocation and death. COPD is the fourth-leading cause of death in the United States, with 118,000 people succumbing to it annually. However, by quitting smoking you significantly decrease your risk for developing all smoking-related diseases, including COPD.

The principles included in this chapter are not meant to scare you. They are included to make you think about the dangers of smoking—and to get you to personalize the statistics you must ignore when you continue to smoke.

PRINCIPLE #40

Know that smoking increases your risk of dying from lung cancer by 90 percent.

You may be shocked to learn the statistical odds of actually dying from lung cancer. According to the U.S. Department of Health and Human Services, approximately 90 percent of lung cancer deaths in men and nearly 80 percent in women are caused by smoking. Additionally, by continuing to smoke, men are 23 times more likely to die from lung cancer than non-smokers, while female smokers are about 13 times more likely. Clearly, smoking stacks the odds against you. Quitting now allows you to significantly reduce your chances of developing lung cancer.

Principle #41

Picture having to lug around an oxygen tank in order to breathe.

---- ❋ ----

When the beautiful Ava Gardner died at the age of 67, her last words were, "I'm so tired." It is no wonder the famed actress was exhausted. She was a lifetime smoker who suffered from emphysema, a disease that causes lungs to lose their elasticity. Loss of elasticity prevents the small airways within the lungs from remaining inflated during exhalation, which causes air to become trapped. Symptoms associated with this brutal disease include shortness of breath, hyperventilating, and an expanding chest. Those who suffer from emphysema eventually require supplemental oxygen to breathe. And, as Gardner sadly discovered, there is no cure for emphysema once it develops.

Principle #42

Understand that smoking causes *many* types of cancer.

※

Though lung cancer is the most well-known cancer associated with smoking, there are many lesser-known cancers that are also caused by smoking. They include oral, pharynx, larynx, esophageal, cervix, kidney, lung, pancreas, stomach, and bladder cancers. You may wonder how smoking affects organs so far from the mouth and lungs. Smoking causes carcinogens to accumulate in organ tissue throughout the body, increasing the likelihood of developing cancer in many different areas. And when it comes to the bladder, smoking causes toxins to accumulate in urine, which can damage the bladder lining and increase the risk of cancer. There truly is no area of the body that is not harmed by continuing to smoke.

PRINCIPLE #43

Know that smoking jeopardizes your heart.

———————— ❊ ————————

Since harmful chemicals attach to and travel with your red blood cells, the heart is the clearinghouse for all toxins in your body. The heart is, thus, particularly susceptible to damage from smoking. According to the American Heart Association (AHA), smoking makes a person 2 to 3 times more likely to have a fatal heart attack. Smokers who are overweight, have high cholesterol, and/or high blood pressure face an even greater chance of dying from a heart attack. Smoking also causes blood to clot more than is healthy and threatens the success of recovery after bypass surgery. These are all compelling reasons to give your heart a break from the toxicity of smoking.

Principle #44

Learn how smoking affects female reproductive health.

✳

Smoking is a particularly destructive habit for women. Not only are women susceptible to cancer and heart disease but their ability to have healthy children may be compromised. According to the 2004 Surgeon General's Report on Women and Smoking, women who smoke may experience irregular or missed periods and be at risk for early menopause. Smoking also increases a woman's chances for delayed conception, infertility, and spontaneous abortions. Smoking has this effect because of the way it alters hormone production in the body. If you want to increase your chances of having children, give smoking the boot.

Principle #45

Bone up on the link between smoking and osteoporosis.

— ✳ —

More than 20 years ago, researchers discovered a link between smoking and osteoporosis, particularly in women. Today, the National Osteoporosis Foundation (NOF) estimates the disease affects 10 million Americans, 80 percent of whom are women. Female smokers should know that smoking decreases estrogen levels and inhibits calcium absorption. This combination causes bones to weaken over time, resulting in frequent fractures that take longer to heal. The same holds true for the 2 million men with osteoporosis. However, by quitting smoking, exercising, and increasing calcium intake, NOF says the risk of developing osteoporosis for both sexes can be greatly decreased.

Principle #46

Think about it: Smoking deprives your brain of oxygen.

———————————— ✳ ————————————

Most people who smoke don't realize that cigarettes can cause brain damage; once they do know they tend to throw their pack straight in the trash. Indeed, smoking wreaks havoc on your body's command center. With each puff, carbon monoxide is transferred into your blood, which decreases the amount of oxygen your red blood cells can transport to your brain. Eventually, depriving your brain of oxygen leads to "lethargy, confusion, and difficulty in thinking," according to the San Francisco-based organization Smoking Cessation. Hence, lifetime smokers can expect to suffer from memory loss and have difficulty concentrating.

Principle #47

Make an appointment to see your doctor… *again.*

With the countless health problems related to smoking, it is no wonder smokers spend more time at the doctor than non-smokers. A study in the *International Journal of Epidemiology* found that male smokers in Japan incurred 33 percent more medical costs for in-patient care per month than non-smokers. In the U.S., the Centers for Disease Control estimates that smokers are responsible for $75 billion annually in smoking-related medical costs—or $3,561 per smoking adult. This is because smokers often suffer from chronic respiratory infections, take longer to heal from illnesses and surgeries, and have compromised immune systems.

Principle #48

Take your mouth off the front lines.

In the war smoking wages on your health, your mouth is on the front lines. Besides increasing your risk of lip, tongue, and mouth cancer, smoking also makes smokers 6 times more likely to develop gum disease than non-smokers. Over time, smoking causes chronic inflammation that forces gums to recede. This exposes the buried portions of teeth, which may cause them to loosen or fall out. However, a 2005 study conducted by dental researchers at the University of Newcastle in the United Kingdom discovered that 20 percent of participants who quit smoking saw a significant improvement in their gum health over a 12-month period compared to those who continued to smoke.

Principle #49

Expect to become tasteless.

— ❋ —

For many smokers, an after-dinner cigarette is as important and enjoyable as dessert—some smokers may actually prefer their cigarette to a dish of ice cream or a piece of pie. Sadly, this indulgence may cause a smoker to have a tasteless meal in the not-too-distant future. Research has consistently shown that smoking harms a person's ability to taste and smell. For example, the American Academy of Otolaryngology has found that the harmful chemicals in cigarette smoke "impairs the ability to identify odors and diminishes the sense of taste." In addition, a 2007 study published in *Alcoholism: Clinical & Experimental Research* found that women with a family history of alcoholism who smoked had decreased sensitivity to sweets. Life is sweet—don't you want to taste it?

PRINCIPLE #50

Usher in ulcers by continuing to smoke.

— ❋ —

One of the more painful conditions that develop from smoking is ulcers. Your stomach is protected by a mucus layer that prevents powerful digestive acids from damaging it. However, smoking damages this lining. This creates open sores, or peptic ulcers. Smokers are further at risk for ulcers because nicotine actually enhances the amount and concentration of stomach acid. Ulcers are extremely painful and get worse the more you smoke. As famed gastroenterologist Dr. Sara Murray Jordan once put it, "Smoking with an ulcer is like pouring gasoline on a burning house." Worse, ulcers in smokers take longer to heal thanks to a compromised immune system and the continuous flow of caustic stomach acids over the ulcer. Avoid developing one at all costs.

Principle #51

Know the link between smoking and Sudden Infant Death Syndrome (SIDS).

───────────── ✳ ─────────────

Smoking while pregnant has consequences that reach beyond your health or even that of your unborn baby. Researchers have discovered a link between Sudden Infant Death Syndrome (SIDS) and mothers who smoke while pregnant. In a 2008 study, biologists at McMaster University learned that as a result of nicotine exposure in utero, some babies born to mothers who smoked while pregnant are unable to self-regulate their breathing while asleep. This makes them more prone to SIDS, in which babies die in their crib. The SIDS-smoking link is just one of a million compelling reasons not to smoke while pregnant.

PRINCIPLE #52

Understand the presence of nicotine in your breast milk is toxic for your baby.

———————————— ❊ ————————————

If you gave up smoking while pregnant but are dying for a cigarette now that baby is born, consider the following before you light up: Nicotine, like alcohol and caffeine, can seep into breast milk. And when you consider the average newborn weighs between 7 and 9 pounds, ingesting nicotine can be devastating. Babycenter.com reports that breast-fed babies of mothers who smoke a pack a day or more experience vomiting, diarrhea, rapid heart rate, and restlessness. When you weigh the risks (to your baby) versus the rewards (satisfying your craving), you should be able to see that lighting up is simply not worth it.

PRINCIPLE #53

Think smoking is swell?
So do your joints.

—————————— ✳ ——————————

Smoking cigarettes can contribute to rheumatoid arthritis (RA), an autoimmune disease that causes painful joint inflammation. RA can be particularly bad in smokers who already have some form of arthritis. Researchers at the American College of Rheumatology released a 2006 study that found that smokers double their risk for developing a severe case of RA. Scientists believe the link between smoking and RA is a result of a smoker's compromised immune system, but quitting smoking can help. The study found that former smokers had a decreased risk, and that women who had quit 10 years or more before the study had no increased risk for RA at all.

Principle #54

Smoke and look 10 years older!

— ✳ —

It is ironic that so many Americans continue to smoke despite living in a youth-obsessed culture. Smoking ravages the body, producing many visible signs of premature aging, such as leathery skin, wrinkles, yellowing of the teeth and fingers, a graying complexion, and the breakdown of collagen, a substance that gives skin its elasticity. In fact, in one study researchers were able to detect deep-set wrinkles under a microscope on the faces of smokers who were just 20 years old. Despite the severity of smoking's effect on appearance, it is possible to halt smoking-related aging by quitting. Indeed, living out the rest of your life as a non-smoker prevents further damage to skin and hair and also increases the odds that you will eat better and exercise more often.

PRINCIPLE #55

Ask yourself if you want scaly, red patches on your skin.

❋

Some smokers will not quit unless an appeal is made to their vanity. If this tactic works on you, then consider that, as a smoker, you are at risk for developing a severe case of *psoriasis*, a skin disease caused by inflammation that produces red, scaly patches. In a study of psoriasis patients, Dr. Cristina Fortes discovered that participants who smoked a pack of cigarettes or more per day had double the risk of severe psoriasis than people who smoke 10 or less cigarettes a day. Fortes also found that the severity of psoriasis was proportional to the number of cigarettes smoked. So quit smoking to protect your beautiful, clear skin.

Principle #56

Consider whether you want to die prematurely.

———————————— ✳ ————————————

It is time to ask the big question all smokers avoid—are you prepared to die prematurely? In addition to the horrific health consequences of smoking, the bottom line is that this habit kills. A report issued by the Centers for Disease Control (CDC) estimates that smoking decreases lifespan by about 10 years. In other words, if your natural life expectancy is 86, you are likely to die at 76 if you smoke. When you consider that the Bureau of Labor Statistics categorizes those 85 and older as the fastest-growing segment of the population, it becomes terrifyingly clear that dying at 76 is truly premature.

OVERCOMING THE
FEAR OF QUITTING

Quitting smoking is often less about learning to live without cigarettes and more about learning to control your *fear* of living without them. As with many other challenges, it is a person's fear of the situation—fear of failure, fear of change—that is most daunting. Countless poets, philosophers, statesmen, and artists have quipped on the debilitating quality of fear. Usman B. Asif may have put it best when he said, "Fear is a darkroom in which negatives develop." In other words, fear breeds negative emotions, habits, and experiences, and thus must be overcome to triumph at any endeavor, including quitting smoking.

The best way to confront your fear of quitting smoking is to get to the heart of what terrifies you. Are you scared you will be a less happy person? Are you frightened of changing your habits, schedules, and acquaintances? Or, perhaps the part about quitting smoking that terrifies you most is the possibility that you will fail. If so, you share something with 17.5 percent of female smokers and 10.7 percent of male smokers. A recent study found that for these people, "fear of failure" was why they had not stopped smoking, even though they wanted to quit.

While it is a realistic concern, the fear of failure should never stop you from achieving what you want. Facing your fear of quitting exposes the myths and realities of your fear and also empowers you to do the self-exploration necessary for this kind of lifestyle change. Nine times out of 10 you will discover that your fears are grossly exaggerated. For example, you may be afraid to quit smoking because you worry you will lose your mind without nicotine. But the truth is, you will probably be a calmer, less agitated person. These common exaggerations do more harm to your psyche than you can imagine. As the sacred Jewish text the Talmud tells us, "If you add to the truth, you subtract from it." When we do what we fear, we almost always come out the winners. It is truly never too late to overcome your fears about quitting smoking, as the following principles will highlight.

Principle #57

Put your fears in check.

———————— ❈ ————————

Unchecked fear is much like a runaway snowball—it spins out of control, gaining size and momentum until it is a scary, unstoppable force. Keeping your fears in check, therefore, is key to beating them. To keep fears about quitting in check, evaluate if they are grounded in reality. For example, one common fear smokers have about quitting is that they will gain weight (as 41 percent of female smokers say they fear). This fear is easily wiped out by vowing to incorporate 30 minutes of exercises a few times a week into your cessation program. Allowing the fear of weight gain to prevent you from quitting is akin to avoiding travel because you are afraid your plane will crash—you can eventually get where you want to be if you put your fears in check.

Principle #58

Use affirmations to remind yourself you are capable of quitting.

———————————— ❋ ————————————

While it is natural to be anxious about quitting smoking, negative self-talk that includes, "I can't do this," or "It's too late to quit," sends a message that you do not trust your ability to succeed. Though it may technically be true at this moment, if you truly want to succeed you have to train your brain to trust your resolve to quit. Metaphysical guru Louise L. Hay recommends the following affirmation for such anxiety: "I love and approve of myself and I trust in the process of life." Repeating this or a similar affirmation builds self-confidence and floods your mind with the message, "I can handle whatever life throws at me—including quitting smoking."

PRINCIPLE #59

Chip away at your fear—literally.

❋

As with any large project, quitting smoking becomes more manageable and less daunting when broken down into smaller bits. One way to break your fear of quitting into smaller bits is to represent it as a physical object that you can actually chip away at. There are many ways to make manifest what fear looks like—for example, you might represent the fear of doing your morning commute without a cigarette as a ball of clay. Squish and manipulating the clay while saying, "I am in charge of my fear. I give it shape. I am bigger than it is." By maneuvering the clay's shape and size, while repeating this phrase, you physically and mentally take charge of your fear and chip away at it.

Principle #60

Use relaxation techniques to prepare for situations that make you want to smoke.

✳

A German proverb states, "Fear makes the wolf bigger than he is." Indeed, fear can turn a kitten into a snarling mountain lion, if you let it. As you prepare to quit smoking, tame fear by relaxing your mind and body. Practicing relaxation techniques for just 20 minutes a day will put you into what Dr. Herbert Benson of the Benson Institute for Mind-Body Medicine describes as the "relaxation response state of being." His research indicates that regular deep breathing and meditation establish a stable baseline from which you become able to put fear into perspective. The relaxation response state equips you to get through stressful situations without a cigarette.

PRINCIPLE #61

Don't use fear to justify your habit.

— ❊ —

For some of us, worrying can become an addiction. We obsess about one thing or another, giving an endless supply of energy to negative thoughts and barriers. These barriers—"I've been smoking for too long to quit" or, "Quitting smoking would prevent me from performing well at my job"—become justifications for why a smoker *has* to continue smoking. When you feel yourself reaching for a justification, think: "Stop!" Internally yelling this interrupts thoughts that need limiting. It also gives you space to insert positive messages such as, "I'm excited about who I might be as a non-smoker" or, "I will be the inspiration for everyone at work to quit."

PRINCIPLE #62

Know that everyone who has ever quit was afraid to at some point.

———————————— ❄ ————————————

Giving up smoking requires months, even years, of hard work and maintenance. Such a lifestyle overhaul naturally causes anxiety. Take comfort in the knowledge that you share your fear of quitting with every single person who has ever quit. The difference between you and them is that they have conquered their fear—and now it is your turn. Remember what Dr. Martin Luther King, Jr. once said: "Normal fear protects us; abnormal fear paralyses us. Normal fear motivates us to improve our individual and collective welfare; abnormal fear constantly poisons and distorts our inner lives. Our problem is not to be rid of fear but, rather to harness and master it."

Principle #63

Don't set your quitting clock by fear.

—— ❋ ——

If you have based your timeline for quitting on your fear of doing so, you are dooming yourself to failure before you even start. Get fear out of your plan for quitting. Start by making a list of your fears. Start with the biggest one and work your way down. Next to each fear, write down how many times you have actually seen this fear come to fruition. If you cannot come up with any examples, cross the fear off your list. Deem that particular fear unfounded, and let it go. Finally, make a deal with yourself that each time you remove a fear from your list, you move one day closer to your quit date. By letting go of unfounded fears you remove the misguided perception that life without cigarettes is an impossible dream.

PRINCIPLE #64

Plan to quit—and succeed.

— ✳ —

Sometimes, the only way to dispel fear and succeed at your endeavor is to come up with a plan for how to execute what you are afraid of doing. Instead of waiting to be ready sometime in the future, make a clear plan of action right now for quitting smoking. This proactive step refocuses fear into preparedness and puts you in control of fear instead of it being in control of you. Indeed, planning for how to deal with stress, disappointment, boredom, and anxiety gives you a "field-guide" to refer to when you feel lost without cigarettes. For as William Arthur Ward, author of *Fountains of Faith*, wisely pointed out, "Men never plan to be failures; they simply fail to plan to be successful."

Principle #65

When you can't execute your plan, go with the flow.

❋

Though having a plan in place for quitting smoking is important, you must also accept there will be some situations you simply cannot plan for. Thus, making room for setbacks in your plan gives you "coping elasticity." For example, learning how to survive when you are stuck in traffic without your quit aids is possible when you stop looking for a way out. Instead of panicking, give yourself over to the stop-and-go flow of traffic. Sing along to the radio, recite a poem, take deep breaths, and repeat the following affirmation: "Life is an ocean. I ride its waves. I go with the flow." This calming incantation releases you from trying to control your uncontrollable environment.

Principle #66

Don't go it alone.

--- ❊ ---

Novelist C.S. Lewis was onto something when he wisely wrote, "Friendship is born at that moment when one person says to another, 'What! You too? I thought I was the only one!'" Indeed, nothing makes a person feel strong and comfortable like being in good, relatable company. To avoid fear from paralyzing your effort to quit smoking, reach out to others. Friends and family will likely jump at the chance to help you quit. The best kind of support, however, is someone who personally knows the agony and elation of the quitting process. If you can't find a tangible quit buddy, turn to the Internet. There are dozens of online support groups, chat rooms, and message boards where you can get support and offer it to others in the same position.

Preparing to Quit

NFL Super Bowl champion Emmitt Smith knew something about having to thoroughly prepare in order to reach his goals. In 1993, he was the only running back ever to win a Super Bowl championship, the NFL Rushing Crown, the NFL Most Valuable Player award, and the Super Bowl Most Valuable Player award all in the same season. When asked about his tremendous success in an interview, Smith replied, "For me, winning isn't something that happens suddenly on the field when the whistle blows and the crowds roar. Winning is something that builds physically and mentally every day that you train and every night that you dream."

As you prepare to quit smoking, let Smith's philosophy be an inspiration to you. Smith's winning performance was a result of the hard work he did before game day. So too will your perseverance over your nicotine addiction come about as the result of serious, consistent, and intentional preparation.

Preparing to quit smoking means formulating a plan that deals with both your mental and physical addiction to cigarettes. If you wait until you are faced with a challenge, it may be too late. But preparing in advance for how you will deal with challenges when they arise gives you an advantage over your addiction. In fact, preparing for both the physical and emotional challenges of quitting smoking *before* tossing your cigarettes in the trash can mean the difference between quitting for *good* and quitting for *now*.

The first part of preparing to quit requires you to set manageable goals. These goals should be individual and depend on how much you smoke and your reasons for quitting. They should also be realistic and specific. Examples include deciding to cut down by a certain number of cigarettes per day and choosing a quit date. The second part of preparing to quit requires you to anticipate smoking triggers and have responses and alternatives ready to go. This may include making difficult choices, such as avoiding certain people you know will make you want to smoke. Once all of these components are in place, you are prepared for Quit Day and to give up smoking for good!

Principle #67

Set a quit date right now.

❋

Work will always be stressful, bills are always due, the kids are always late or loud, and the housework never seems to get done. Therefore, your quit date must be established firmly, in spite of the rest of your life. Life won't stop happening to give you time to gently usher in change. So choose a date right now, and vow to keep it, no matter what else comes up. To choose a date, give yourself time, but not too much time. A month or two from today is perfect; 6 months from today is too long and will cause you to lose momentum. Put a large red "Q" on all your calendars so your quit date exists both at home and at work. And, finally, commit to the Q! Allowing Quit Day to come and go without action will damage your resolve, so choose a day and stick to it.

Principle #68

Take advantage of positive public pressure to quit smoking.

---- ❋ ----

If you were to tell just 5 family members, friends, or coworkers about your decision to stop smoking, it is likely you would be met with cheers of excitement, congratulations, and encouragement. That's because quitting smoking, unlike other challenges, is a widely supported goal, especially now that the dangers of smoking and secondhand smoke are so well-known. Take advantage of this aspect of your challenge as you prepare to quit. Tell just 5 people about your decision to quit smoking and you have likely just enlisted 5 personal cheerleaders. Look to these people to keep you accountable to your goal when you face challenges or are tempted to smoke.

Principle #69

Create a blueprint for quitting.

—— ✳ ——

Napoleon Hill, author of the highly influential book, *Think and Grow Rich*, once wrote, "Every well-built house started in the form of a definite purpose plus a definite plan in the nature of a set of blueprints." Indeed, our houses are only as strong as we planned them to be and the same is true about our success at quitting smoking. To build a solid foundation for your cessation plan, start to anticipate now what needs you might have while you are quitting. What healthy snacks are you going to reach for instead of a cigarette? How are you going to cope if a stressful situation befalls you while you are quitting? Create strategies for dealing with these situations now so you do not have to scramble when in the midst of it.

Principle #70

Talk to your doctor about kicking the habit.

———————— ❋ ————————

Consulting with your doctor fulfills a few different needs during the smoking cessation prep period. First, it adds another witness to your public declaration to quit. It also serves to hold you accountable, since you will see your doctor at least once a year for your annual physical. But, perhaps most satisfying is that your doctor will be able to give you feedback over time on how your health has improved as a result of quitting smoking. He or she will be able to tell you how your airways have cleared and are capable of taking in more air, or congratulate you on losing a few pounds as a result of your ability to breathe easier while exercising. Don't skip this critical prep step.

Principle #71

Find a quit buddy.

———— ✳ ————

Having a quit buddy is a tried-and-true strategy for kicking the habit. It is comforting, motivating, and creates a small "former smoker" community base. Also, statistics from a 2008 study published in the *New England Journal of Medicine* show it is more likely that you will quit if you are surrounded by others who also quit. The study found that when one spouse quit, the odds of their partner continuing to smoke fell by 67 percent. Similarly, when friends of study participants quit, smoking among their friends fell by 36 percent. Researchers also found that quitting smoking at work caused coworkers' smoking to decrease by 34 percent. Have a quit buddy lined up in advance for your quitting effort.

Principle #72

Throw away smoking paraphernalia.

———————— ✳ ————————

Ashtrays, lighters, matches, cigarettes, pipes, and other smoking paraphernalia are remnants from your smoking life and therefore constitute temptations. They must be removed from your home if you are to successfully quit smoking. If not, their presence will sit in the back of your mind like a neon sign flashing, "Smoke!" It is especially important during the first few weeks of your cessation program to get rid of these items. Most important is to throw out the emergency smoke stash that you keep in the back of your drawer or in the glove compartment of your car. Extinguish the possibility of a smoking slipup by doing an honest sweep and ridding your environment of items that will tempt you to smoke.

PRINCIPLE #73

Begin an exercise program.

❋

Starting an exercise program before you are about to give up smoking may sound like torture! But doing just 20 to 30 minutes of physical activity a day will help prepare you for Quit Day. Beginning an exercise program now establishes a new routine and adds structure to your day. This will become an important substitute once your time is no longer guided by a smoking schedule. Indeed, the American Lung Association (ALA) recommends at least 30 minutes of vigorous exercise (which can be broken up into 10-minute intervals throughout the day) while in the process of quitting smoking. The ALA's rationale? Exercise and smoking are incompatible; doing one, therefore, will make it much less appealing for you to do the other.

Principle #74

Identify your "I'm done" moment and write it down.

— ❋ —

Former smokers often have a collection of experiences that support one main "I'm done" moment. For some, the main reason is a frightening health experience, such as a heart attack or cancer diagnosis. Others quit because their children or partner ask them to. Whatever your "I'm done" moment was, write it down. Add other reasons when they occur to you. For example, if your main reason was, "I'm done smoking because I can't keep up with my toddler," you might also add that you want to see your child graduate from college or to be around for your grandchildren. Writing down these reasons should reveal a connection to your big "I'm done" moment.

Principle #75

Start weaning yourself away from triggers.

———————————— ✳ ————————————

If you are like most smokers, you probably engage in other behaviors that enhance your enjoyment of smoking, such as drinking, eating certain foods, spending time with certain people, or savoring a cigarette for a certain time of the day. In fact, what you consume while smoking, the locations in which you smoke, and the people you smoke with have all become triggers that tell you it's cigarette time. Thus, to remove temptation, you must avoid the triggers—at least until you feel confident that you have quit for good. Weaning yourself away from these triggers now will decrease the intensity of your smoking urges on Quit Day and beyond.

PRINCIPLE #76

Enter into a quit contract with yourself.

———————————— ❋ ————————————

Bind yourself to quit smoking by signing a cessation contract with yourself. The language of the contract should be simple, but clear. It should include the date you plan to quit, a few reasons for quitting, that you understand the challenges you face, and that you plan to succeed. Then, sign and date the contract and ask a friend or family member to sign as a witness. Your witness should be someone you care for deeply and do not want to disappoint. Some people ask their spouse or one of their children to sign, feeling more accountable if it is a family member. Whomever you choose to sign the contract, know that it is an effective tool used by Oprah Winfrey to lose weight many years ago!

Principle #77

Join a smoking-cessation program.

————————— ✳ —————————

Some people just know they cannot quit on their own. If you are one of these folks, consider joining a smoking-cessation program. There are countless such groups, including Nicotine Anonymous and other private and community organizations. Their programs, combined with groups, books, DVDs, medications, and nicotine-replacement aids more than double your chance of quitting smoking and staying quit. According to the American Heart Association, smoking-cessation programs are especially effective for people who smoke 25 or more cigarettes a day, so heavy smokers should definitely seek help from a program. Quitting smoking is often a group effort. Don't worry if you need a little bit of help—there is plenty out there.

Principle #78

Fill an "idea book" with activities to replace smoking.

———————— ❊ ————————

The biggest question smokers want answered when deciding whether to quit is, "What will I do if I'm *not* smoking?" This is a fair question, and is why the American Lung Association suggests brainstorming replacement activities in advance. In fact, we think you should go so far as to create a non-smoking "idea book" in which you write down ideas for how to fill the time normally spent smoking. Examples include doing a crossword, chewing gum, sipping a smoothie, eating carrots, jogging in place, giving the dog a bath, reorganizing the closet, or shuffling cards. Carry the book with you and refer to it when needed. Finally, add to it when you feel inspired.

PRINCIPLE #79

Get therapy for depression and anger.

———————————— ❊ ————————————

A study of male and female smokers found that 63.1 percent of women and 55 percent of men reported they were worried about how they would manage their stress without cigarettes. Quitting smoking when you harbor unaddressed anger, stress, or depression seriously compromises your chance for success. When you are depressed or angry, you start your cessation program from an unstable place. Your anger becomes like a fuse that is prone to going off at any time. Therefore, during your preparation period, seek therapy for any problems you have with stress, anger, or depression. Working through difficult issues before adding the challenge of quitting smoking is the best way to position yourself for success.

PRINCIPLE #80

Read testimonials on the Internet by other successful quitters.

※

Internet-based encouragement comes in many forms, but perhaps most instructive are Websites that feature testimonials from people who have quit smoking. In preparation for your Quit Day, read at least 10 testimonials. In them you will find tips, tricks, ideas, and honest accounts of the challenges people just like you face as they become non-smokers. Read a sampling of people, because a person who quit 2 days ago will have a different testimonial from one who has been smoke-free for 25 years. Take the best from all of them to create your own brand of cessation wisdom—and remember to write your own testimonial so that others may learn from you.

PRINCIPLE #81

Know what to expect during the first few weeks.

※

There's no use pretending the first few days and weeks after Quit Day will not be difficult. You will face a number of physical and emotional challenges, but knowing what to expect will demystify the experience and allow you to prepare to deal with it. Know going in that for the first few weeks you are likely to experience fatigue, headaches, dizziness, coughing, sore throat, nasal drip, anxiety, difficulty sleeping, trouble concentrating, and the constant temptation to smoke in order to relieve these symptoms. This is why cessation experts agree that having a plan in place to deal with these symptoms is absolutely critical to your success.

Principle #82

Repeat, "I am a non-smoker" any time doubt crowds your thoughts.

— ❉ —

One of the best ways to prepare to quit smoking is to train your mind to think of yourself as a non-smoker—even before Quit Day. Thinking this way puts you in a powerful frame of mind. Tell yourself, "I am a non-smoker. I do not need cigarettes." Do this and by the time Quit Day arrives you will have already started the difficult task of changing your mind set from smoker to non-smoker. As the classic author John Milton once wrote, "The mind is its own place, and in itself, can make heaven of Hell, and a hell of Heaven." For the unprepared, quitting cigarettes truly is a hell, so let your mind help you turn the situation into a peaceful, easy heaven.

Tapering Off

Actress Barbara Kelly once said, "I tried to stop smoking cigarettes by telling myself I just didn't want to smoke, but I didn't believe myself." Like Kelly, many smokers are unable to quit because their desire for a cigarette is so strong. Going cold turkey often worsens this problem because it heightens the desire for a cigarette. This is why many ex-smokers find success in tapering down their cigarette habit before they quit altogether.

The effectiveness of tapering off is best appreciated by comparing the effort to climbing a mountain. From the foot of the mountain, the peak looks incredibly far away. If someone were to say you had until tomorrow to get to the top, you'd probably head back to your house. Even if you were to be transported to the top of the mountain, the sudden change in pressure and altitude would render you breathless and nauseous. Quitting cold turkey is very much like this scenario—it makes a person sick, overwhelmed, and unprepared for the effort. Imagine, however, being only 100 feet from the mountain's summit—you could probably muster your energy to make it to the top. Next, imagine being just 100 feet away from the place at which you are 100 feet from the summit ... and so on. Tapering off is like this approach to mountain climbing—it prepares you so thoroughly, step by step, for your large goal that you hardly feel like you are accomplishing anything harder than the sum of its parts.

Make no mistake, however: tapering off requires as much discipline and commitment as quitting cold turkey does. At a certain point, you still must stop smoking. But by cutting down the amount of nicotine you take in over time, you will be less addicted by the time you quit. Though it is true that tapering off is not for everyone, it does have its place for those who do it correctly. To learn how to taper off your cigarette intake to successfully quit smoking, use the following simple principles. They are full of ideas that encourage discipline with action-oriented steps that even the heaviest smoker will find useful.

Principle #83

Switch brands.

— ❈ —

Smokers cultivate their habit to be as satisfying as possible, and this includes developing a loyalty to their favorite brand of cigarettes. One way to lose your taste for cigarettes is to switch to a different brand that has less nicotine and tar. However, this is not license to smoke more cigarettes in a day! Remember, your goal is to taper down to zero cigarettes. The point of switching brands is to make smoking less appealing, while reducing the amount of nicotine your body needs. Therefore, if you alter the filter, take deeper drags, or smoke more than you normally would you are defeating the purpose of this tapering technique. So, only switch brands if you are truly ready to commit to the weaning process, because it can backfire if you are careless.

Principle #84

Alter your smoking schedule.

The National Institutes of Health (NIH) recommends hitting snooze on your automatic smoking clock by consciously choosing when you smoke. Some ways to do this are to delay your first cigarette of the day by 1 hour. As you get within a week or two of your quit date, delay it by an additional 5 minutes each day. Also, practice smoking cigarettes only when you *really* want them. Check in with yourself after lunch and ask yourself if you "need" a cigarette. If the answer is, "I could probably live without one," go back to work until you cannot go another minute without smoking. By extending the time in between cigarettes, you slowly dismantle your automatic smoking clock while reducing the amount of nicotine your body needs.

PRINCIPLE #85

Choose a "last call" time of night for having a cigarette.

❊

Once you take control of your smoking schedule you learn you do not "need" as many cigarettes as you thought you did. Setting boundaries for when you allow yourself to smoke will highlight this point even further. After 2 or 3 days of delaying your first cigarette of the day by 1 hour, choose a time at night that is "last call" for smoking. Last call should be at least 1 hour before bed and, like with the morning-delay program, bump back last call by 5 minutes each day as you get within 1 to 2 weeks of your quit date. This extends the greatest length of time between cigarettes—while you are asleep—and trains your body to need less nicotine.

Principle #86

Smoke less every day until Quit Day.

———————— ✳ ————————

Cutting down the number of cigarettes you smoke until Quit Day is a mathematical exercise that many smokers prefer. Its appeal is that it delays the proverbial "pulling off the Band-Aid"—or quitting cold turkey. However, it is important to have a handle on your habit before engaging in this technique. For optimal success, know exactly how many cigarettes you smoke daily and have a rough idea of when your Quit Day is before you enact this plan. Smokers of 20 or more cigarettes daily should smoke 1 less cigarette every day over a period of a month, leveling off at around 7 cigarettes per day. Once down to 7 cigarettes a day, commit to a Quit Day. You have so dramatically reduced your habit by this point, you are in an excellent position to quit completely.

Principle #87

Make a tapering-off schedule and stick to it.

— ✳ —

The tapering-off method helps you get control over your habit, reduce the amount of nicotine your body craves, and gives you time to adjust to giving up cigarettes altogether. But without an end date in mind, you are at risk for continuing to smoke less instead of actually quitting. Though it is better to smoke less than more, there is no "safe" number of cigarettes. A study published in *Tobacco Control* found that men and women who smoked between 1 and 4 cigarettes a day nearly tripled their risk of dying from heart disease. So as you reduce your cigarette consumption, stick to your schedule and remain 100 percent committed to your Quit Day.

Principle #88

Don't smoke in comfortable situations.

———————————————— ✳ ————————————————

In *The Picture of Dorian Gray,* Oscar Wilde wrote, "A cigarette is the perfect type of a perfect pleasure. It is exquisite, and it leaves one unsatisfied. What more can one want?" Indeed, the pleasure-need-pleasure cycle is among the most compelling reasons smokers have for not quitting. But it is possible to alter the pleasure of smoking by changing how you smoke. For example, don't allow yourself to smoke while sitting down. Avoid pairing a cigarette with a glass of wine or scotch. Such changes reduce the smoking experience down to just you and the cigarette. While in this stripped-down state, focus on the unpleasantness of standing in the cold or how you look in the mirror, alone. Internalizing these images trains your brain to view smoking as a lonely and cold habit not to be enjoyed.

Principle #89

Make smoking inconvenient.

❋

An old riddle asks, "What is a smoker without cigarettes?" The answer—a non-smoker! Train yourself to be a non-smoker by keeping cigarettes and other smoking paraphernalia in inconvenient locations. For example, keep cigarettes in a shoebox under the bed and store matches and lighters in different locations throughout the house—including the freezer. For as one saying goes, "The best way to stop smoking is to carry wet matches." In addition to hiding your stash, don't bring your cigarettes to work with you. Leave them in the car or at home so you have to work to get them. Each minute you spend looking for your cigarettes and for something to light them with increases your time tolerance between cigarettes.

Principle #90

Buy a pack, not a carton.

※

We live in a buy-in-bulk society. With stores like Costco, BJ's, and Sam's Club, and with the increasing price of cigarettes, it is no wonder smokers have gotten in on the act of stocking up. However, this is one habit you must cease immediately in order to successfully taper off your smoking habit. Only buy cigarettes one pack at a time. Likewise, never allow yourself to purchase the next pack until you have finished the last cigarette in your current pack. Several studies have shown that people are more economical with how many cigarettes they smoke—that is, they smoke fewer of them and less often—when they only have a few left, as opposed to knowing there are several packs stored away in a drawer at home.

Principle #91

Never finish a cigarette.

— ❊ —

It may seem odd, but putting out a cigarette before you finish it is a powerful tapering technique. When used in combination with a tapering-off schedule, buying packs instead of cartons, and not smoking when it will be most pleasurable, discarding half-smoked cigarettes is a valuable lesson for smokers. It proves you don't need to smoke an entire cigarette to feel satiated. Like the other tips, it also serves to wean your body from high levels of nicotine. In addition to half-smoking your cigarettes, the NIH recommends that smokers trying to quit collect their butts in a large glass jar, and keep it visible. The visual impact of hundreds of half-smoked, crushed butts is very unpleasant and functions as a reminder of how disgusting smoking is, and why you should quit.

PRINCIPLE #92

Pick a number from 1 to 10.

※

If you want your tapering plan to have a solid structure, try the following: select a number of cigarettes you plan to smoke during the day in advance. Then, have only that many on hand. For example, if you decide to smoke 8 cigarettes on Tuesday, Wednesday, and Thursday, only take 8 with you when you leave the house on those mornings. As you choose when to smoke each cigarette, be mindful of what time it is and how many cigarettes you have left. Even if you know there are more cigarettes at home, stamp it into your brain that you are only allowed to smoke 8 today. As Quit Day approaches, reduce the number of cigarettes you are permitted to best position yourself to quit for good.

Principle #93

Swap gum for smokes
for just one full day.

❄

Once you are within a few days of Quit Day, practice going 24 hours without smoking. Curb your craving by swapping cigarettes with nicotine gum, a patch, or another quitting aid. This dry run helps prepare you for what it will feel like on Quit Day but has the cushion of knowing you are allowed to smoke the next day. And who knows? If this practice goes well, you may decide not to smoke the next day either. Expect to feel a range of emotions, from, "This isn't as hard as I thought" to, "I can't do this!" Above all, know that whatever you feel is perfectly valid and keep yourself calm by remembering you are just trying it out for one day.

DEVELOPING WILLPOWER

Quitting smoking requires developing self-discipline so that you have the willpower to stay on track when temptations to smoke arise. There is no greater example of self-discipline than the Indian leader Mahatma Gandhi, who once said, "Strength does not come from physical capacity. It comes from an indomitable will." Of course, most smokers have trouble asserting their will over temptation, which is usually how they started smoking in the first place. One reason willpower is so difficult for smokers to cultivate is that it starts with making the decision to quit—and then sticking to it. Some smokers find it challenging to make decisions in general, while others have trouble following through with them. Either way, if you want to quit smoking, you must learn to stick to your cessation program by employing willpower.

Since willpower is often associated with making choices that cause one to feel deprived, it is helpful to reframe your thinking. Instead of feeling like you are missing out on cigarettes, picture a long, rich life that begins on Quit Day. Obviously, quitting will not be without its challenges, but focusing on missing out on smoking, instead of filling up with life, diminishes your will to resist smoking. In addition, boost willpower by living a disciplined lifestyle in which you combat laziness, procrastination, and immediate gratification. This work will benefit you in all aspects of your life. Indeed, practicing self-restraint is character-building and rewarding for many reasons.

One important component of willpower is saying "no," which is usually the least enjoyable part of quitting anything for people. Yet for such a little word, "no" packs a lot of punch and is critical to master. For example, if your friends are going for happy hour after work and you will be tempted to smoke—skip it. Exercising self-discipline in these early days of quitting shortens the length of time you must skip regular activities to avoid temptation. To get there sooner, use the following principles to boost your will to quit—and remember that quitting smoking starts with a choice but is sustained by willpower.

PRINCIPLE #94

Don't procrastinate.

— ❊ —

Once you decide to quit smoking, do not wait another minute to act or you run the risk of depleting your will to quit. Even if you just sit down with a calendar to plot out your tapering-off schedule or to choose your Quit Day, do something immediately. Your success depends on action with momentum behind it. As author Eva Young once warned, "To think too long about doing a thing often becomes its undoing." With this in mind, know that each step you take toward quitting fuels your will to give up smoking and increases your desire to be disciplined about never smoking again. Don't wait for the perfect time to quit, because there is never going to be a better time than right now. In fact, think of now as the *only* time.

Principle #95

Be enthusiastic about quitting.

❋

In Arlington National Cemetery, there is a sculpture dedicated to the Seabees, men and women of naval construction battalions. The inscription on the sculpture reads, "With willing hearts and skillful hands, the difficult we do at once; the impossible takes a bit longer." Think of this epitaph as you develop your willpower and use it to regard willpower as a machine that requires fuel to function. Now imagine that your enthusiasm for quitting is fuel with the highest efficiency rating. In other words, it is your job to drive your enthusiasm for quitting through the roof so there is no shortage of fuel for your willpower. Positive messages like these steer you away from the feeling that you are making a great sacrifice, which is important to the preservation of your will to quit.

Principle #96

Know your desired outcome.

———————— ✳ ————————

Those who climb Mount Everest face unimaginable weather, geographical challenges, and even death. Yet dozens of people attempt the climb every year because they know, despite the obstacles, exactly where they plan to end up—on top of the world! This analogy is useful for smokers who feel as though they are facing a mountain of unknown difficulties and a fear that they are not up to the task. Visualize your goal of becoming a non-smoker, because having clarity about your desired outcome allows you to focus on getting there, and focus leads to commitment and willpower. Understand that your path may not always be clear, but as long as you know where you want to end up, you are capable of getting there.

Principle #97

Don't stop until you can commit 100 percent of yourself to quitting smoking.

❊

When breaking your addiction to smoking, you must be 100 percent committed with a singular focus—to quit completely. Otherwise, you will constantly feel deprived and be tempted to smoke. "One foot in the door, one foot out" behavior weakens the foundation of your overall goal, not to mention your will to quit. As spiritual guru Sri Chimoy points out, "If part of you still subconsciously harkens after the bad habit, your focus will be split and you will not be able to generate the necessary willpower." Thus, it is better to put your Quit Date off a few weeks until you are able to be 100-percent committed.

Principle #98

Live healthily across the board.

—— ✴ ——

For most smokers, cigarettes are not the only unhealthy vice they've allowed into their lives. Cigarette addiction usually goes hand in hand with an overall unhealthy lifestyle that can include excessive alcohol consumption, high caffeine intake, a diet based on processed and junk foods, and avoidance of exercise. Though quitting smoking is the most important change to make right now, changing these other habits at the same time will support your cessation program because they, too, require self-discipline. Moreover, committing to a healthier lifestyle requires planning and high self-regard—vital components of willpower. Finally, once you have broken your addiction to cigarettes, you will find it feels natural and logical to improve your health in other areas, too.

Principle #99

Build up your willpower by achieving smaller victories.

—— ❊ ——

Nothing breeds success like success! By setting and achieving several smaller goals before Quit Day, you build confidence and prove that you are a capable person. For instance, once you see that you are able to produce your desired result—such as smoking 1 less cigarette per day—you won't want to jeopardize that success. Practice setting small goals that you know you can achieve and increase their difficulty as Quit Day nears. Examples include: Don't smoke in your car when you are 30 days from your quit date; half-smoke all cigarettes when you are 15 days from quitting; and donate $1 to charity for every cigarette you smoke the day before you quit.

· PRINCIPLE #100

Stay firmly grounded in the present.

———————————— ✳ ————————————

There is no sense in trying to quit smoking if you start out believing you will fail based on past attempts. Likewise, torturing yourself with the notion of never having another cigarette for the rest of your life is too large a burden to bear at this stage in your quitting effort. Both recalling past failures or looking too far into the future prevents you from concentrating on the present, which is necessary for the newly quit smoker to stay motivated. Remember that your willpower is dependent on how you view your chances of success. With that in mind, be an optimist and believe in the best possible outcome. As 19th century psychologist William James wrote, "Pessimism leads to weakness, optimism to power."

PRINCIPLE #101

Focus on the benefits of quitting.

---- ✳ ----

Staying focused on the benefits of giving up cigarettes reminds you that quitting is worth it—especially since great willpower is required at this early stage to prevent you from smoking. Although it will feel like a tremendous sacrifice to go without cigarettes, you must keep your mind on the positive outcomes quitting will have on your health. Reread chapter 4 in this book for a refresher on how unhealthy smoking is. Then, think of what spiritual guru Sri Chimoy once said: "If we are clear on the benefits then we will work to improve our willpower. If we don't value the benefit of strong willpower we will not improve it." Improving your willpower results from standing by your decision to quit, and viewing this choice positively.

Principle #102

Follow intuition when your thoughts threaten to derail you.

— ❋ —

Intelligent, thinking people often have more trouble quitting smoking than their less-cerebral peers. This may seem odd, but it makes sense when you consider how overthinking a plan can actually delay its enactment. Mulling over every possible withdrawal symptom, challenge, or setback may cause you to throw up your hands in defeat before you ever quit. Therefore, shut off your brain and coast on intuition in the first few weeks of your quitting effort. As English poet Robert Graves once pointed out, "Intuition is the supra-logic that cuts out all the routine processes of thought and leaps straight from the problem to the answer."

Principle #103

Believe you will succeed.

※

The power of the mind is truly astounding. As Henry Ford put it, "If you think you can do it, or you think you can't do it, you are right." Ford knew a little something about willpower—that's how he became the preeminent maker of American automobiles when others doubted his ability. Similarly, the sheer act of doubting or believing you have the willpower to quit smoking makes you correct. Since willpower is a form of positive energy that lets you commit to accomplishing a goal, you must generate enough of it to get through your cessation journey. A strong inner will is crucial for times when you are blinded by the desire for a cigarette.

Principle #104

Find inspiration in unexpected places.

———————————— ✳ ————————————

Would you be surprised to learn that an overweight friend you have not seen in a year has since lost 100 pounds? Your first thought might be, "I didn't think he had it in him!" In fact, your view of him as weak because he was fat is similar to how you view your own willpower to quit smoking. But instead of thinking of your friend or yourself as "fighting weakness," be inspired by humanity's motivation to change and our ability to achieve results. Though losing weight and quitting smoking are not identical, they have much in common. Both require discipline and willpower, so when seeking out inspiration remember to look beyond your own set of circumstances and bond with anyone who has overcome a great obstacle or is in the process of trying.

PRINCIPLE #105

View yourself as a role model.

———————————— ❊ ————————————

Acting as a mentor increases your desire to do your best, ratcheting up willpower and your ability to avoid cigarettes. This is especially important when you consider that according to the Substance Abuse and Mental Health Association (SAMHA), about 1,300 kids under 18 become regular smokers every day. If you are seen smoking by kids, you essentially become an advertisement, even an advocate, of cigarettes. Instead, see yourself as an ambassador for *not* smoking. Psychologist Dr. Phil has described the value of becoming a role model in the following way: "Through your actions, your words, your behavior and your love, you can direct your children toward where you want them to go." This same advice is true of your ability to help others avoid cigarettes.

PRINCIPLE #106

Say "no" to low-consequence situations.

———— ✳ ————

One of the best ways to flex the willpower muscle is to exercise it regularly. So, even before you have officially reached your Quit Day, practice saying "no" when friends or coworkers offer you a cigarette. You are likely to receive surprised looks and perhaps even hear some sarcastic comments in response. But don't give in! Walking away from low-consequence temptations (i.e., you don't really need the offered cigarette because you have a pack in your car) is good practice for when you actually quit. It also prepares those around you for the change that is coming. Each time you walk away from an offered cigarette, you demonstrate your willpower to resist the urge to smoke in social situations.

DEALING WITH WITHDRAWAL

Dr. Thomas H. Brandon and his team of researchers from the H. Lee Moffitt Cancer Center and Research Institute made an interesting discovery while studying nicotine withdrawal in smokers. They found that pack-a-day-smokers experience anxiety, anger, sadness, and difficulty concentrating within an hour of having a cigarette. This is why heavy smokers consume about 1 cigarette every 40 minutes—to counteract these feelings.

What does this mean for you in your effort to quit smoking? It means that, as a moderate or heavy smoker, it is very likely you are already familiar with what withdrawal feels like. You've been through it before in small doses—it is not a foreign experience to you. This is very important for you to know as you quit smoking. A poll undertaken by the American Cancer Society (ACS) found that a whopping 70 to 90 percent of smokers say their *only* reason for not quitting smoking is because they are afraid to face the withdrawal.

Although the fear of withdrawal often discourages people from quitting, Brandon and his team found that even the most severe withdrawal symptoms peak within about 3 days of a person's final cigarette. After that, they become more mild and cease completely after about 2 to 3 weeks. Focus on getting through this initial period by comparing it to other activities that would fly by in 3 days, or for which 3 days would not be enough time. The hardest part of your withdrawal period will be shorter than the average vacation, the average conference, or the average workweek. In fact, the period you have to make it through is just about the same length as the animal with the shortest lifespan on Earth. This is the *gastrotrich*, a tiny aquatic animal, which lives for just 3 short days.

Author Paolo Coelho wrote, "Tell your heart that the fear of suffering is worse than the suffering itself." Truthfully, getting through the withdrawal period is worth it, and often not as hard as you have imagined. Use the following simple principles to get you over this much-feared hump.

PRINCIPLE #107

Count your way through withdrawal.

——————————— ✳ ———————————

An old saying goes, "Patience is counting down without blasting off." Experiencing withdrawal will take extreme patience, and it is OK to use the classic tool of counting to get through it. When you feel the urge for a cigarette coming on, do slow counts of *1 Mississippi, 2 Mississippi*, all the way up until you reach 100. Feel free to modify your count as you need to. Some smokers like to count the parts of their body they are making healthier: *1 Healthy Pink Lungs, 2 Healthy Pink Lungs*, etc. Whatever you choose to count, by the time you are done adding it up, you will have gotten through the moment of temptation.

PRINCIPLE #108

Prepare yourself for emotional withdrawal.

Although our bodies move through the physical symptoms of withdrawal in 3 days or less, it often takes our minds much longer to catch up. Indeed, the hardest part of withdrawal you will face is not likely to be physical withdrawal but emotional withdrawal from your lifestyle as a smoker. Surviving emotional withdrawal means avoiding the places and scenarios in which you would normally light up. If your commute feels too empty without a cigarette, try the bus for a few weeks. If your coffee feels incomplete when not paired with a cigarette, switch to tea for a while. Train yourself to make new associations that do not involve cigarettes.

Principle #109

Never let yourself go.

✳

The withdrawal period is trying enough for the new non-smoker, but failing to take care of your basic needs can make it much worse. A lapse in self-care triggers a different need in all of us, but the most common ones are hunger, exhaustion, boredom, and loneliness. Should any of these needs elevate to a state of desperation, you become likely to succumb to withdrawal and reach for a cigarette. Therefore, figure out which state is most threatening to you and never let yourself get there. Keep snacks on-hand to stave off hunger; take on extra work if you are worried about getting too bored. Make sure to get plenty of sleep while you are in the early stages of quitting, and surround yourself with supportive company.

Principle #110

Drop and do 10!

———————— ✳ ————————

When you are in the throes of a craving, the last thing you want to do is 25 sit-ups. However, a study published in the journal *Addiction* found that short bursts of exercise reduced participants' cravings for nicotine and prolonged the amount of time they were able to go between cigarettes. The studies showed that even just a brisk 5-minute walk was enough to head off smoking, indicating that longer exercise sessions— though helpful—were not necessary. In addition, reviewers noted that exercise is effective in curbing the urge smoke because it "curbs stress, improves mood, and spurs the release of brain chemicals that may override nicotine cravings." When your body is screaming for a cigarette, drop and do 10 pushups to send that craving into remission!

PRINCIPLE #111

Stay hydrated.

———————— ❋ ————————

The human body is made up of more than 50 percent water, and everyday activities, such as sweating during exercise, cause the body to dehydrate The fluid lost must be replenished—especially during the withdrawal period when your kidneys use water to flush leftover toxins from cigarettes out of your body. Drinking 8 glasses of water each day—more when it is hot or you are very active—will also prevent you from getting dehydrated, which can cause severe changes in your body chemistry as well as prevent your kidneys from doing their job. Plus, dehydration exacerbates withdrawal symptoms such as headaches and irritability. Therefore, choose water over sugary sodas or juices to quench your thirst while in withdrawal.

Principle #112

Reduce your caffeine intake.

❊

According to Johns Hopkins University School of Medicine, 80 to 90 percent of North American adults and more than 165 million Americans report using caffeine regularly. Smokers make up a large percentage of caffeine consumers. But large amounts of caffeine cause people to develop headaches, feel irritable, get dehydrated, and all-around crash—symptoms you are already combatting during withdrawal. Therefore, as nicotine leaves your system, help your body out by not giving it another drug to withdraw from. Seek a milder boost from tea or light, healthy snacks that keep your blood-sugar levels steady. Also, avoid heavy, greasy foods that will make you feel sluggish. Caffeine is definitely not your friend while you are going through withdrawal.

PRINCIPLE #113

Temporarily cut back on drinking.

━━━━━━━━━━━━━━━ ✳ ━━━━━━━━━━━━━━━

While in withdrawal, it is OK to enjoy a glass of wine with dinner or a cold beer at a barbecue—but don't over do it. Alcohol impairs your ability to think clearly, and you are likely to succumb to nicotine cravings while under the influence. Furthermore, alcohol prevents your liver from breaking down sugar and makes your kidneys sluggish, and you need these organs working optimally to rid your body of toxins. Also, alcohol is a depressant, and you will already be prone to depression in the first few weeks of quitting. For all of these reasons, it is best to avoid alcohol during this time. It can be daunting to kick two vices at once, though, so tell yourself you can have that glass of wine once you get to a more stable place in your cessation program.

Principle #114

Tap the millions of ex-smokers at your disposal.

❋

An astonishing 46 million Americans count themselves as ex-smokers. With numbers like these, it is possible that smokers trying to quit have one of the largest support networks in the world at their disposal! You can find these ex-smokers, and other newly quit smokers suffering through withdrawal, at a multitude of organizations, hospitals, and online and in-person communities that offer free support groups. Find a group near you through the American Heart Association, the American Lung Association, the American Cancer Society, Nicotine Anonymous, the National Cancer Institute, and the Smoking Cessation Leadership Center.

Principle #115

Use nicotine-replacement therapy.

― ✳ ―

Nicotine-replacement therapy (NRT) has been shown to double the chances of successfully quitting smoking when used properly and with other methods of support, such as cessation programs, quit groups, online chat rooms, family and friends, and quit buddies. That's why the American Cancer Society recommends using NRT in conjunction with these other efforts to ease the physical symptoms of withdrawal. Examples of NRT include nicotine patches, gums, nasal sprays, inhalers, and lozenges. There is no evidence to support that one type of aid is better than another. It is a matter of preference, depending on your particular needs. Choose one and have it on-hand for when your cravings strike.

Principle #116

Get your squeeze on.

—— ❊ ——

When you first quit, the risk of relapse is high, in part, due to the stress of managing withdrawal symptoms. One way to deal with that stress is to carry around a tennis ball so you have an object on which to take out your frustration. When you feel the urge to smoke or become irritable, angry, or weepy, squeeze the tennis ball with all your might. Throw it against the wall if you have to! In fact, throw it across the room so you have to repeatedly go get it; then after you pick it up, squeeze it as if you mean to crush it. Do whatever it takes to get pent-up energy out. Channeling energy normally curbed by smoking through another activity is an effective way to get through the darkest part of the withdrawal period.

Principle #117

Call 1-800-QUIT-NOW for immediate support.

———————— ※ ————————

The U.S. Department of Health and Human Services runs a free program for the public called 1-800-QUIT-NOW. This is a valuable service with an easy-to-remember number for people in all stages of quitting. Callers are able to speak with a counselor who will provide cessation support as well as information on coping with withdrawal symptoms and coordinating a quit plan. Trained counselors are equipped with the most up-to-date information regarding nicotine-replacement therapy and coping strategies for cravings and slipups. This a free government-sponsored program that is available 24 hours a day—take advantage of it in your time of need.

PRINCIPLE #118

Deal with withdrawal by getting crafty.

— ❋ —

Taking up a new hobby is an excellent way to distract yourself from the pangs of withdrawal. Hobbies that require the use of your hands are particularly effective. Sewing, painting, playing music, and crafts are all excellent choices. In fact, Elizabeth Zimmerman, a famed knitter, author, and host of a PBS series on knitting once said, "Knit on, with confidence and hope, through all crises." Indeed, Zimmerman was so adept at knitting that she was able to knit while riding on the back of her husband's motorcycle! Though you may never be able to knit under such extreme circumstances, surely you will be able to use knitting and other crafty hobbies to navigate through the ups and downs of the withdrawal period.

PRINCIPLE #119

Use essential oils to manage withdrawal symptoms.

———————————— ✳ ————————————

Aromatherapy has been used for centuries by the Chinese, Egyptian, and Indian people to aid in digestion, ease nausea, boost the immune system, and promote relaxation. It works by causing smell receptors to send a message to the brain's limbic system, which controls mood and emotion. The National Cancer Institute reports that essential oils may reduce nausea and anxiety for cancer patients undergoing chemotherapy. Since nausea and anxiety are common symptoms of nicotine withdrawal, inhaling lavender, bergamot, sandalwood, peppermint, cardamom, ginger, or spearmint oil may significantly reduce these adverse side effects.

Principle #120

Hang out in the non-smoking section—even in your own home.

※

Where there is smoke, there are smokers, so as you fight through the withdrawal period it is important that you stick to non-smoking zones. Seeking out places where smoking is not allowed is one way to use behavior modification to control your urge to light up and distract you from your withdrawal symptoms. The good news is that non-smoking sections are all around you. As of 2008, 14 states had banned smoking in bars or restaurants, or both, and others had legislation proposing a ban. Movie theaters are another great smoke-free place in which to seek refuge. And, of course, make your home and car non-smoking, even for your guests.

Principle #121

Build, organize, or clean something.

———————————————— ✳ ————————————————

Avert cravings by throwing yourself into an all-consuming endeavor, such as a building, cleaning, or organizing project. This will distract you from—and delay—satisfying the craving. Reorganize your bathroom, construct a birdhouse, put together a model train set, or paint the house. Organize old photos, clean out the garage, or do the most thorough spring cleaning you've ever done, even if it is winter. These projects are time-consuming, require use of both hands, demand your concentration, and produce tangible outcomes as a reward. However, it is important to have these projects and materials on-hand so that when a craving strikes you can head straight to the birdhouse and start hammering.

Principle #122

Brush your teeth every few hours.

— ❋ —

The National Heart, Lung, and Blood Institute and the American Dental Association are among the many national organizations that recommend you avoid nicotine cravings by brushing your teeth several times a day, or at least after every meal. Studies show that people who consistently brush their teeth throughout the day are deterred from smoking by having fresh, clean breath more so than those who brush just twice a day. In addition, this extra brushing helps remove yellow residue leftover from your smoking days and allows your gums to recover from their years under smoky assault. Flossing regularly and using an antimicrobial mouthwash in addition to brushing will also cause your dentist to rejoice at your next checkup.

Principle #123

Look into Nicotine Anonymous meetings.

If faith is a strong influence in your life, consider joining Nicotine Anonymous. This program is modeled after Alcoholics Anonymous and follows 12 steps to an addiction-free lifestyle. You start by admitting that you are powerless over nicotine and that your life has become unmanageable. By the time you reach the sixth step, you will admit, "We're entirely ready to have God remove all these defects of character," including the continued craving for nicotine. For many, this relieves the guilt and pressure of not only quitting but having ever become addicted. Meetings are a great place to find support from others with a severe nicotine addiction.

Principle #124

Stay organized with lists and an updated calendar of events.

———————————— ✳ ————————————

You may notice that shortly after your Quit Day, you find yourself having an uncharacteristically hard time concentrating on things. This is common and is the result of nicotine withdrawal. As your body deals with this temporary setback, help yourself out by planning ahead and staying organized. Keep an updated calendar where you write down commitments. Have a pad and pen with you at all times to write down important information, or get in the habit of emailing yourself reminders. Keeping tasks in order will prevent you from giving in to the urge to smoke when withdrawal symptoms make you unable to concentrate.

Principle #125

Realize that falling asleep may take some work.

❉

Quitting smoking suddenly shoves normal activities, such as going to sleep, into a new light. Many newly quit smokers complain of insomnia, which is interesting, since nicotine is a stimulant, not a relaxant. Regardless, insomnia is a cruel, yet temporary, existence. While getting 8 hours of sleep may be impossible right now, take steps to increase your sleeping hours. Reduce caffeine intake, take a warm bath before bed, ask your partner for a 10-minute massage, sip herbal tea, drink warm milk with honey and nutmeg, avoid alcohol, get regular exercise, meditate for 30 minutes before bed, and try getting up half an hour earlier.

PRINCIPLE #126

Visit a hypnotherapist.

---- ❊ ----

There is no question the physical symptoms of nicotine withdrawal are exacerbated by the emotional stress of managing cravings and other side effects. Finding ways to cope with all components of withdrawal at the same time is important. One way is to get hypnotized by a licensed hypnotherapist. The concentrated state of relaxation of hypnosis allows the therapist to reprogram your subconscious mind to believe that you are a non-smoker—and, of course, non-smokers do not crave cigarettes. Suggestions given while in this state, such as, "You no longer crave nicotine," and "You will sleep well tonight," may decrease symptoms while increasing your rate of success by as much as 66 percent, according to the American Society of Clinical Hypnosis.

Principle #127

Don't spin out of control—
there is relief for dizziness.

❊

Within the first few days of quitting, many people experience dizziness. This is from an increase in oxygen to your brain—which is a good thing! But it can take your body time to get used to this extra oxygen, so take care when dizziness strikes. Sit down immediately and take several deep breaths, or lie down and put an ice pack on the back of your neck while breathing deeply. Also, drink lots of cool water. If dizziness is accompanied by nausea, drink ginger tea, chomp on ginger chews, or put grated ginger on a slice of lemon and inhale. And for daily maintenance, take a vitamin B6 supplement to support brain health and balance.

PRINCIPLE #128

Seek treatment for depression.

❈

Nicotine is a stimulant. When you smoked, you were given steady bursts of a chemical high. Now that these boosts are gone, you may find yourself feeling uncharacteristically down in the dumps. This feeling should pass within a few weeks, but if it doesn't, you may be depressed. Depression requires treatment, such as therapy and/or medication. If you become unable to perform daily activities; avoid friends, family, and social functions; have trouble performing at work; or are unable to meet your basic needs, seek help. Treating depression is an important component in managing not only your nicotine-withdrawal symptoms but also in staying quit from cigarettes for good.

Eating a Non-Smoking Diet

When smokers learn that diet impacts their ability to successfully quit smoking, their first thought is often, "As if quitting smoking isn't hard enough! Now I have to watch what I eat, too?" The short answer is "yes," but it should not be too difficult to make some minor adjustments to give major support to your cessation efforts. The extent to which you find eating a non-smoking diet difficult depends on your current eating habits. But wherever your habits, tastes, and preferences fall on the spectrum, know that you can remove much of the misery and temptation of quitting smoking by eating a nutrient-rich, balanced diet.

Several prominent studies have confirmed that certain foods and drinks are triggers for smoking relapse because they enhance the enjoyment of cigarettes. A study conducted by Dr. F. Joseph McClernon and his team of researchers for Duke University, for example, found that 70 percent of smokers report meat, alcohol, and caffeinated beverages made cigarettes taste better. Forty five percent of participants said dairy products, juice, water, fruits, and vegetables made cigarettes taste worse. Of these findings, McClernon said, "The conventional wisdom is that cigarette addiction is all about the nicotine... But we are learning more and more it is also about sensory effects like the taste and the smell and the visual experience and the habitual routines of smoking. The taste effects are important."

Eating a non-smoking diet, therefore, involves foods that don't pair well with smoking. In addition, sticking to a nutritionally sound diet prevents excessive weight gain— a common side effect of the quitting process and a grave concern for ex-smokers. Examples of healthy ways to deal with nicotine cravings without piling on pounds are drinking a glass of low-fat milk when you would normally smoke, or orally fixating on carrot and celery sticks instead of a cigarette. For more tips on how to use nutrition to quit smoking—and for ideas to plan your non-smoking diet— consult the following simple principles.

PRINCIPLE #129

Track your eating habits for 3 days.

———————— ❋ ————————

Like smoking, people tend to eat without thinking. But by tracking meals and snacks for 3 days you force yourself to become conscious of your eating habits. For this exercise, make 3 columns on 3 pages in a notebook. Label the columns, "What," "When," and "Why." Be diligent and write down every morsel of food, the time it was consumed, and your reason for eating it. An example of an entry is: "What—potato chips, chocolate bar, and cola; When—2 p.m.; Why—I was bored and wanted a cigarette." After 3 days, a pattern will emerge about what you crave, when, and why. Identifying this pattern empowers you to anticipate weak points during the day so you are prepared to handle cravings in healthier ways.

Principle #130

Fill up on fiber-rich foods.

❋

Eating foods high in fiber keeps you full longer, preventing overeating. And besides eliminating hunger, fiber-rich foods reverse health problems from years of unhealthy living by reducing cholesterol, decreasing the risk of developing colon cancer, easing constipation, and lowering the amount of insulin required to process sugar. The FDA recommends eating 25 to 30 grams of fiber daily, yet most Americans only consume between 10 and 15 grams, and that number may be even lower for smokers who tend to have less-healthy eating habits. Fiber-rich foods to incorporate in your diet include whole grain breads and cereals, beans, spinach, berries, nuts, brown rice, potatoes with skin, peas, oranges, apples with skin, and dried fruits such as prunes.

PRINCIPLE #131

Defeat free-radicals by adding antioxidants to your diet.

———————————— ✳ ————————————

Your body produces normal levels of harmful molecules called free-radicals in response to diet and metabolism. But smoking cigarettes dramatically increases their production, making you susceptible to premature aging, heart and lung disease, cancer, and other diseases. According to Dr. Dean Ornish of the Preventative Medicine Research Institute, antioxidants help remove free-radicals and decrease your risk for developing disease. Foods rich in vitamins A, C, and E—such as citrus, peppers, broccoli, green leafy vegetables, artichokes, strawberries, nuts, seeds, and others—scavenge free radicals, and can prevent and even reverse smoking-related disease.

Principle #132

Avoid acidic beverages if you use
nicotine-replacement products.

❋

People who smoke more than a pack a day will most benefit
from nicotine-replacement therapy (NRT). However, diet plays
an important role in the efficacy, so avoid sabotaging it with
unhealthy food and drink choices. According to the American
Lung Association (ALA), acidic beverages like coffee and soda
may prevent your body from absorbing the nicotine in NRT
products. Replacing coffee and soda with herbal teas and plain
or flavored water lets you support both your NRT and a new,
healthier lifestyle. The ALA also recommends ceasing to eat
or drink 15 minutes before and after chewing NRT gum to
allow maximum nicotine absorption.

Principle #133

Keep healthy snacks as close as you did your pack of smokes.

---※---

Actress Mae West once quipped, "I never worry about diets. The only carrots that interest me are the number you get in a diamond." Many smokers are similarly disinterested in carrots the vegetable. But having ready-to-go, crunchy, healthy snacks on hand is an excellent way to curb oral cravings without packing on pounds. Wash, cut, and store snacks like carrots, celery, grapes, jicama, bell peppers, and apples in single-serving containers. To satisfy salt cravings, buy baked chips, low-salt pretzels, nuts, air-popped popcorn, rice cakes, and graham crackers. Anticipating cravings and preparing for them helps fight the urge to smoke and keeps you slim.

PRINCIPLE #134

Find healthy alternatives to junk food.

—————————— ❊ ——————————

Picking healthy alternatives to your favorite junk foods is a great way to prevent gaining weight after quitting smoking. It's easy to eat a diet that satisfies salty and sweet cravings without driving up the needle on the scale. One example is enjoying a smoothie instead of a milkshake. Smoothies are great for breakfast and snacks and include vitamin-packed fruit. To boost protein and calcium add low-fat yogurt, milk, or soy milk. Also, many places that serve smoothies offer vitamin packets for little additional cost. Other examples of healthy substitutes include baked potatoes instead of fries, reduced-fat cheeses, balsamic vinegar and olive oil instead of sugary salad dressings, veggie burgers instead of hamburgers, and whole grain bread instead of white bread.

PRINCIPLE #135

Help your immune system bounce back.

———————— ✳ ————————

Smokers are often shocked to learn that smoking cigarettes has weakened their immune systems. According to the *Health Science Report*, damage inflicted on the immune system by smoking is second only to that of chemotherapy. However, like most other smoking-related problems, quitting now significantly reduces the problem. The immune system can be stimulated by eating nutrient-rich foods such as yogurt, mushrooms, citrus, onions, tomatoes, garlic, spinach, pumpkin, sweet potatoes, canola and olive oils, oysters, crab, turkey, and squash. All these foods contain immuno-boosting levels of beta-carotene, vitamin C, vitamin E, and zinc. In addition, these foods are low in fat and calories, so regular consumption will not cause you to gain weight.

Principle #136

Don't inhale smoke—or your food.

————————— ✳ —————————

In their determination to refrain from smoking, quitters often stuff their mouths with another substance: food. Overeating while quitting smoking is the main reason why ex-smokers gain weight, and gaining weight is a main reason why smokers put off quitting entirely. A recent poll found that 41.1 percent of female smokers and 14.6 percent of male smokers reported a "fear of gaining weight" as the reason they do not quit smoking. An easy way to avoid this fate is by chewing your food slowly and deliberately. This gives your digestive system time to activate, which stimulates the more efficient breakdown of food. It takes about 20 minutes for your stomach to send signals to your brain that you are full, so that you can avoid overeating.

Principle #137

Think before you eat.

※

No diet or smoking-cessation program in the world will work unless you are willing to think before you act. While this primarily applies to thinking before you reach for a cigarette, it also applies to thinking before you reach for your next snack. The greatest threat to your non-smoking diet is allowing yourself to eat mindlessly. Mahatma Gandhi once advised, "Those who know how to think need no teachers." In this spirit, let your body rhythm teach you when to eat and how much by taking a few minutes to evaluate whether you are truly hungry before you eat. Noticing how often you eat when you are not hungry and then coming up with alternative activities will dramatically cut down on calorie consumption as you navigate the difficult waters of nicotine withdrawal.

PRINCIPLE #138

Stock your kitchen before Quit Day.

※

The best way to combat smoking cessation-related cravings is to be prepared to deal with them. Stocking your kitchen with healthy, ready-to-eat snacks is part of laying this groundwork. Make a comprehensive shopping list and hit the market before Quit Day. Stock the fridge with lots of crunchy produce, low-fat dairy products, and fruit. Fill the cabinets with healthy edibles like dark chocolate, creamy soups, and whole grain breads and cereals. Gearing up for Quit Day by having lots of food options should prevent you from hopping in your car at 11 p.m. to hit the nearest fast-food drive-thru. Stock your kitchen in the spirit of what the inventor Henry Ford once said: "Before everything else, getting ready is the secret to success."

Principle #139

Set realistic dietary goals.

— ✳ —

Lofty goals such as, "I will never eat fast-food again," are unrealistic and therefore frustratingly unreachable, especially in this initial quitting period. Be specific about your dietary goals as they relate to your quitting effort, and don't put too much pressure on yourself. For example, if you want to avoid replacing cigarettes with sugar, limit yourself to a couple sugary treats per week. Then, write acceptable treats on a calendar, choosing the days on which you will eat them. Have only the pre-decided number of sugary snacks in the house and after each has been eaten, cross it off the calendar. Sticking to your non-smoking diet means crafting reasonable goals you can live with.

Principle #140

Stick to recommended portion sizes.

— ❋ —

Comedian Woody Allen, known for his curmudgeonly attitude, once remarked, "The food here is terrible—and the portions are too small!" Allen's joke rings especially true to people who have recently quit smoking. Even though food tastes less satisfying than a cigarette, they still want to eat too much of it. In addition, American portion sizes have dramatically increased over the past 40 years, as New York University researchers discovered in a recent study. Avoid piling on pounds during your cessation period by paying attention to the portion sizes listed on labels—even when cravings tempt you to eat more. When eating out, try eating half the food on your plate and getting the rest to-go.

Principle #141

A dairy product a day keeps the cigarettes away.

—— ❊ ——

Several studies on quitting smoking have revealed that dairy products—in particular, yogurt, cottage cheese, and milk—have a repellent effect on smokers. A study conducted by Dr. F. Joseph McClernon and his team of researchers at Duke University, for example, found that 45 percent of smokers put dairy products on a list of foods that they claimed made cigarettes taste worse. Make sure to stock your fridge with these items and eat them when you feel the urge for a cigarette coming on. Plus, these foods are a good source of calcium, lean protein, and healthy vitamins that will be beneficial to you as you rebuild a healthy body.

PRINCIPLE #142

Avoid red meat.

─────────── ❊ ───────────

Eating red meat poses a double-whammy for smokers—it enhances the desire to smoke and increases the risk for developing heart disease and some cancers, which smokers are already prone to. This is especially true for women. A study conducted by Harvard Medical School found that women who ate 1.5 servings of red meat per day doubled their risk for developing breast cancer. Furthermore, the study revealed that women who regularly ate red meat also tended to be smokers and overweight. The connection between red meat and the desire for cigarettes is unexplained, but it is clear that red meat has no place in the non-smoker's quitting diet. Instead of hamburgers and steaks, try turkey, chicken, salmon, or substitute a grilled veggie burger.

Principle #143

Learn which foods are cigarette-repellent.

—————————— ❊ ——————————

As a smoker, you were accustomed to choosing foods and drinks that complemented, even enhanced, the satisfaction you got from smoking a cigarette. But as a new non-smoker you must think exactly the opposite. When you want to smoke, think, "What can I eat or drink that would be absolutely terrible with a cigarette?" Oranges, lettuce, tofu, apples, carrots, cucumbers, oatmeal, lemonade, milk, orange juice, and water have all been shown to have a cigarette-repellent quality. Fill your kitchen with these items and leave out foods and drinks that trigger the desire for cigarettes, such as coffee, soda, alcohol, red meat, fried foods, and commercially baked goods.

PRINCIPLE #144

Know that if you do gain weight, you will probably lose it soon.

※

Despite your efforts to adopt a non-smoking diet, it is possible that you might gain a few pounds while you are quitting. If so, don't panic—it is likely this weight gain is temporary, as a study published in the *Journal of Consulting and Clinical Psychology* found. Researchers evaluated changes in diet, activity levels, and weight gain among subjects who quit smoking. They found that after 2 weeks of quitting cigarettes, subjects exhibited a significant increase in calorie intake. But by week 26, caloric intake for a significant number of the ex-smokers was equal to or even less than when they quit. Have patience, and you will stay both trim and smoke-free for life.

CALMING YOURSELF
WITHOUT CIGARETTES

Ask any smoker why they puff, and you will probably get an answer that relates to relaxation. In fact, the National Cancer Institute reports that stress management is one reason most people smoke. A survey of hundreds of male and female smokers discovered that 63.1 percent of women and 55 percent of men reported that the number one reason they chose not to quit cigarettes was because they were worried about how they would manage their stress without a smoke. Indeed, the prospect of calming oneself without a cigarette is a valid and common concern for newly quit smokers.

The good news is that countless studies have shown that relaxation exercises such as deep breathing, yoga, and meditation decrease the severity of withdrawal symptoms, establish a calmer baseline for dealing with crises, and improve overall health and immune functioning that has been damaged by years of smoking. Therefore, it is in your best interest to carve out 20 minutes each day to decompress and calm your nerves. Making time for relaxation also has tremendous health benefits. According to the Mayo Clinic, relaxation techniques lower blood pressure; slow your heart rate; increase blood flow and oxygen; and reduce muscle tension, backaches, and headaches.Moreover, regularly doing yoga and meditating has been shown to boost the immune system while reducing the number of colds and flu. Clearly, there are many compelling reasons to begin a relaxation regimen.

English author Cyril Connolly once wrote, "The secret of success is to be in harmony with existence, to be always calm, to let each wave of life wash us a little farther up the shore." Achieving such a tranquil state is certainly easier said than done for ex-smokers fighting through nicotine cravings and withdrawal, but is possible with a little bit of knowledge and effort. The following principles will teach you how to quiet yourself without the aid of a cigarette and, in that sense, offer you a true, genuine calm.

Principle #145

Be quiet.

———— ❄ ————

Quitting smoking is an irritating experience on its own. But when you add outside annoyances like the constant noise of television, radio, traffic, and car alarms, chances are your blood pressure will be through the roof by the day's end. The organization Noise Off: The Citizens Coalition Against Noise Pollution has found that exposure to noise pollution causes hearing loss, stress, hypertension, increased blood pressure, and headaches. And since quitting smoking may temporarily lead to some of these symptoms in itself, it is important for new ex-smokers to make time for quiet. With this in mind, try sitting in a quiet room with soft lighting for 15 to 20 minutes in the evening. Note how this practice lowers your heart rate and allows you to wind down for bed.

Principle #146

Remember to laugh!

—— ❋ ——

You may find very little to laugh about in the early days of quitting smoking, but laughter is an often overlooked but effective stress reliever. Dr. Lee Berk and Dr. Stanley Tan of Loma Linda University in California studied the effects of laughter on the immune system and discovered that laughing reduces the stress hormones cortisol and epinephrine, lowers blood pressure, and boosts the immune system by increasing infection-fighting T-cells. In addition, laughter releases endorphins—the body's natural painkiller—and results in a general sense of well-being. So, incorporate laughter into your cessation program. Rent funny movies, visit a comedy club, or spend time with a friend who tells hilarious stories— as long as you are laughing you will not be smoking!

Principle #147

Calm yourself by chanting.

❋

The ancient practice of chanting is useful when struck by an intense need to smoke. It will switch your focus from seeking external solutions to finding inner peace. Chanting using a mantra—a sound you make that creates a certain vibration— will help you focus your energy and strength until your craving has passed. Tsangsar Tulku Rinpoche defined the following 6-syllable mantra used in many Buddhist traditions. They are *Om* (meditation or bliss), *Ma* (patience), *Ni* (discipline), *Pad* (wisdom), *Me* (generosity), and *Hum* (diligence). You may want to choose just one that speaks most to your personality or hum the chant all together as *Om Mani Padme Hum*. You should chant in a droning tone that causes you to feel relaxed yet alert and focused until the urge to smoke is gone.

Principle #148

Touch prayer beads during stressful situations.

———————————— ✳ ————————————

Keep a set of prayer beads with you for quick meditation and calming when you feel as though you might succumb to the temptation to smoke. Rosary beads, Buddhist prayer beads called *malas*, or even string of inexpensive plastic beads will do the trick. Your beads should be accessible to you at all times, including during your commute, at work, while traveling, and, of course, in your home. Whenever stress creeps in, so too will your urge to smoke. Pick up your beads, touch each bead, breathe, and say an affirmation or prayer. Repeat the same affirmation or prayer as you move your fingers over the beads. Continue to do so until you no longer desire a cigarette.

PRINCIPLE #149

Use deep breathing to get into a relaxed state.

※

Most people—particularly smokers—take only shallow breaths. However, slow, deep breaths treat your mind and body to extra oxygen and much-needed release from the stressors of your day. Even taking just one good breath and holding it can give someone a slight, pleasant buzz. After years of smoking, it may be difficult for you to get a good breath at first but, with time, deep breathing will come more naturally. Carve out 5 minutes each day to focus on breathing. Tune out everything out except for the natural rhythm of the rising and falling of your chest and shoulders as you breathe. When faced with the urge to smoke, take deep breaths instead.

Principle #150

Guide your mind away from smoking.

———————— ✳ ————————

A great way to reduce quitting-related stress and nicotine cravings is to make guided imagery (GI) recordings. GI is a relaxation technique in which calming images are described as you listen with your eyes closed while breathing deeply. One popular example of guided imagery is hearing yourself described as a point in the center of a triangle. As you settle into this image, picture the triangle filling with cool, blue light. This image, when delivered in a soothing tone, may reduce anxiety by up to 65 percent. Reducing anxiety will cause you to feel more relaxed overall, which gives you a more stable baseline for dealing with nicotine cravings. It is so relaxing, in fact, that it is recommended that you do not listen to GI recordings while you are driving.

PRINCIPLE #151

Make time for meditation.

────────── ❋ ──────────

Meditation is a proven way to reduce stress and become centered in your identity as a non-smoker. This ancient tradition of concentrating on a particular object or concept will bring relief from smoking withdrawal in as little as 5 minutes. Meditation increases blood flow and slows your heart rate while increasing mind-body awareness. It also reduces anxiety by lowering the levels of lactic acid in the blood. To receive the full benefits of meditation, practice twice a day for 20 to 30 minutes. As you settle into a relaxed posture, simply be aware of your breath and how it feels to breathe in clean air without smoke. Focus on healing your body with breath and allowing pent-up stress and nicotine cravings to flow out of your body with each exhale.

Principle #152

Practice yoga to connect your smoke-free mind with your smoke-free body.

———————— ✳ ————————

The regular practice of yoga offers exceptional support to ex-smokers who require an activity to reduce stress and replace smoking. Yoga relieves stress because it forces you to breathe deeply, which increases blood flow to your limbs and organs, and also decreases blood pressure, helping the body heal from your smoking days. In addition, yoga leaves its practitioners with a sense of calm and inner peace, alleviates stress, and encourages as sense of control and order. As poet Ymber Delecto said of the practice, "Yoga is invigoration in relaxation. Freedom in routine. Confidence through self control. Energy within and energy without."

Principle #153

Take your mind on a journey away from smoking.

———————— ✳ ————————

Journey meditation is a great substitute for smoking. This technique integrates deep breathing with visualization exercises to achieve a state of deep relaxation. If practiced correctly, journey meditation will leave you feeling refreshed and free of the urge to smoke. To practice it, sit comfortably and think of a peaceful place. An isolated mountaintop is an ideal mental destination. Picture yourself resting on warm sandstone, thousands of feet above civilization. Feel the soothing sun as it heats your skin. Hear the wind whistle. Notice the absence of cigarettes, lighters, and ashtrays and watch as your urge to smoke slides away.

Principle #154

Use Tai Chi to improve coping skills.

———————— ❋ ————————

Tai Chi's "meditation in motion" properties have allowed it to evolve into an elegant form of exercise since its inception in 16th-century China. Its increasing popularity around the world is due to its ability to reduce stress, give greater balance, and increase flexibility. In addition, Tai Chi movements are low-impact, which make them appropriate for all fitness levels. Tai Chi is accessible to even the most out-of-shape ex-smokers who wish to improve their physical and emotional health. Indeed, a study published in the *Journal of Behavioral Medicine* discovered that Tai Chi left practitioners with lower levels of depression and stress than those who were sedentary. Since your success depends on managing your emotional response to quitting smoking, it is worth giving Tai Chi a try.

DEALING WITH SETBACKS

Though you should never plan to fail at your attempt to quit smoking, it is important to be prepared for the possibility that setbacks may occur within the first 3 to 6 months. In fact, the American Cancer Society reports that it takes most smokers 5 to 7 tries before being able to quit for good. American writer Mark Twain once put the difficulty of quitting for good in the following way: "To cease smoking is the easiest thing I ever did. I ought to know because I've done it a thousand times." These statistics and ideas are not meant to discourage you, but rather to reassure you that should you light up after Quit Day, you are not alone. Moreover, there are steps you can take to get back on track when you are ready.

Smoking after you quit does more psychological harm than physical. Smoking a cigarette or two is not enough to jumpstart your physical addiction to cigarettes, but it can open the door to becoming mentally or emotionally addicted again.

Should you lapse and have a cigarette, feel disappointment in yourself but avoid spiraling into self-loathing—it is simply an unproductive mind-set. Instead, ask yourself the following questions: *Why did I smoke? Did I enjoy it? What could I have done differently? Am I ready to quit for good this time?* By analyzing the circumstances of your slipup or relapse you give context to what happened without judging. This is how you will learn from your mistakes and move forward.

Once you have a handle on what happened and understand the mistakes you made, your next step is to limit wallowing. Endlessly beating yourself up will not serve any purpose other than to further undermine your self-confidence. At the same time, you must not make excuses for yourself. Avoid letting yourself think, "It's just one cigarette, how much could it matter?" This type of thinking is a highway that leads straight back to smoking.

The trick to dealing with setbacks is to achieve a balance between beating yourself up and letting yourself off the hook. For helpful ideas on how to deal with setbacks, give the following simple principles a try.

PRINCIPLE #155

Give your quitting effort
neither an A nor an F.

———————— ✳ ————————

The Centers for Disease Control (CDC) says that 40 percent of Americans try to quit smoking each year. Of these, less than 1 in 10 will succeed on their first attempt. The reason for this low success rate is obvious—quitting smoking is hard! Unfortunately, newly quit smokers make it harder by putting tremendous "pass or fail" pressure on themselves, instead of allowing room for mistakes and setbacks. As you attempt to quit, give yourself room to get more than just an A or an F for your smoking-cessation effort. Instead, shoot for a B, B+, or an A-. Like millions of other Americans, you aren't perfect—and you don't have to be to become a non-smoker.

PRINCIPLE #156

Don't expect to become a non-smoker overnight.

———————— ❊ ————————

Most people start smoking when they are teenagers and do not decide to quit until they are in their 30s or 40s—or even older. This is a long time to smoke! With such a history, it is impossible to become a non-smoker overnight. As the American Association for Respiratory Care has put it, "It took a while to learn to smoke; it takes a while to learn not to smoke." After all, your task is not as simple as just not smoking cigarettes. It also includes changing your attitude, altering your social habits, retuning your diet, and even making new friends. It is OK if the foundation of your cessation plan suffers a crack now and then—just be confident in your ability to patch it up.

Principle #157

Make sure you get back in the game.

---— ✳ —---

Approximately 75 percent of smokers who want to quit must make more than 1 attempt to kick the habit. Yet each time an ex-smoker slips up and takes a drag from a cigarette, it is a hit to his or her confidence. This small nick has led many ex-smokers to spiral into a full-fledge relapse. It is important to forgive yourself for your smoking indiscretions—no matter how many times they occur—and get right back into your cessation program. As Ralph Waldo Emerson wisely wrote, "Our greatest glory is not in never failing, but in rising up every time we fail." Besides, by viewing mistakes along the way as blips instead of failings, you are less likely to beat yourself up and more likely to try again.

PRINCIPLE #158

Stave off setbacks by being accountable to someone else.

Confess your smoking slipups to another person who is supportive. A study by researchers Nicholas Christakis and James Fowler of the Framingham Heart Study found that being accountable to a partner—preferably someone with quit time under his or her belt—increases a person's chances of successfully quitting smoking by up to 36 percent! As Christakis noted, "Our health behaviors are not just affected by our friends, but by our friend's friend's friend, because behaviors in a network cascade throughout the network." Indeed, the support you exchange with your partner is motivating and rewarding and will help you quit.

Principle #159

Silence your inner critic.

————————— ✳ —————————

Silencing your inner critic is imperative for dealing with smoking setbacks. Beware of the voice in your head that calls you a failure, or the one that deems the tiniest mistake a catastrophe, tempting you to give up completely. Such criticisms undermine your self-esteem, which is a main tool in your arsenal of anti-smoking weapons. You can defeat your inner critic through what anxiety expert Dr. Edmund J. Bourne calls "positive counterstatements." An example of a positive counterstatement is, "Everyone makes mistakes, and I will succeed this time." It is important to establish with your statement that you are not alone, and that you are very capable of becoming a non-smoker, even though you have experienced some setbacks.

PRINCIPLE #160

Learn from your mistakes.

———————————— ❉ ————————————

Henry Ford once said, "A mistake may turn out to be the one thing necessary to a worthwhile achievement." Indeed, sometimes making mistakes actually helps craft the path to quitting smoking for good. Mistakes always contain lessons, even wisdom. Should you make a mistake in your cessation program, think about what you can learn for it. Look upon your mistakes as a stepping stone rather than as a boulder blocking your way. This simple shift in your mind-set clears the way for maneuvering past setbacks, rather than being turned back by them. Besides, making mistakes is human, and learning how to move beyond them is necessary to success in any endeavor.

Principle #161

Don't get cocky.

━━━━━━━━━━━━━━━ ✳ ━━━━━━━━━━━━━━━

While confidence is an asset to your quitting effort, overconfidence is often a liability. Believing that you have defeated your smoking addiction is a sure sign that you are at risk for relapse. Nicotine addiction expert Allen Carr has said, "Smokers who find it easy to stop find it easy to start again." With this in mind, never leave your guard down when it comes to the lure of smoking—not in 6 weeks, 8 months, or even 20 years. If you have been addicted to nicotine, you are always at risk for becoming addicted again. Feeling overconfident in your ex-smoker status may tempt you to believe you can smoke socially or occasionally. But isn't that how you became addicted to smoking in the first place?

PRINCIPLE #162

Realize it may take more than one attempt to quit.

---　❋　---

A Japanese proverb says, "Fall seven times, stand up eight." This saying encapsulates the experience of most American smokers trying to kick their habit. Studies reveal that it takes the average smoker 5 to 7 times before they quit smoking for good. While you must treat your quitting effort as if this is the only time you will ever quit smoking, it is also important to know the statistical odds. Knowing that it may take you several tries to quit should not dissuade you or cause you to put off the effort. Rather, think of it as all the more reason to begin your quitting efforts as soon as possible.

Principle #163

Reach out to your support network.

———————— ❊ ————————

When you decide to quit smoking you have two orders of business—the first is making the decision to quit, and the second is to establish a support network of friends, family, and smoking-cessation experts that you may call upon to help you deal with setbacks. Don't underestimate the impact your support network can have on your quitting effort. A study published in the journal *Health and Education Research* found that women who called a smoking-cessation helpline run by ex-smoking peers had a higher long-term quit rate than those who did not use the helpline. Using quit lines as well as leaning on trusted friends and supportive family members dramatically improves your chances of managing setbacks without giving up on your cessation program all together.

PRINCIPLE #164

If you haven't tried nicotine-replacement aids yet, do so.

❋

According to the American Cancer Society (ACS), only between 5 and 16 percent of ex-smokers are able to go without cigarettes for 6 months without the help of nicotine-replacement therapy (NRT) aids like gums or patches. When they do use these aids, however, they more than double their chances of successfully quitting. If you haven't tried NRT yet, do so now—such aids are likely to stave off setbacks because they slowly wean your body from nicotine. If you have already tried NRT and are still experiencing setbacks, see your doctor. It could be that you are using the aid improperly or need a prescription-level NRT.

PRINCIPLE #165

Know that gaining weight is healthier than quitting smoking.

———————————— ✳ ————————————

One of the top reasons people relapse is because they gain weight after quitting (average is about 2 pounds, though some gain more). Though no one wants to gain weight, experts unanimously agree that smoking just a few cigarettes a day is more harmful to your health than being overweight. And though you may be fed up with weight gain, note that smoking by itself is not enough to drop unwanted pounds. Plus, taking up smoking again puts you in the difficult position of having to quit all over again. Instead of relapsing over weight issues, exercise daily and eat a healthy diet to prevent gaining excessive weight.

Principle #166

Be serious about stress management.

———————— ✳ ————————

The best way to deal with setbacks is to avoid them altogether, and one way to do this is to get serious about managing your stress levels. The American Association of Retired Persons (AARP) warns that reoccurring stress may cause you to get sick more often and have difficulty concentrating, sleeping, and eating. In addition, stress may cause high blood pressure and heart disease as well as anxiety and depression. It is no wonder, then, that unmanaged stress causes ex-smokers to relapse! It it is possible and even easy to lower stress levels through diet, exercise, meditation, staying organized, setting achievable goals, and maintaining close relationships. Indeed, making time to relax each day is necessary for preventing the urge to smoke from becoming too big to handle.

PRINCIPLE #167

Understand that withdrawal symptoms *will* pass.

———————— ✳ ————————

Your withdrawal symptoms will peak about 72 hours after your last cigarette—that's how long it takes for 100 percent of the nicotine to leave your body. This is a difficult time for many ex-smokers, as headaches, dizziness, nausea, and irritability make nicotine cravings very difficult to resist. However, know that smoking even just one puff prolongs the presence of nicotine in your system and the presence of your symptoms. Hang in there through this tough time. Most physical symptoms will subside within 3 days and will be completely gone within 10 to 14 days of quitting.

PRINCIPLE #168

Delay your urge to smoke by 5 minutes when faced with a crisis.

※

New ex-smokers will find that it especially difficult to stay quit when faced with a crisis, such as a death in the family, divorce, unemployment, financial difficulties, a change in your living situation, or the loss of a pet. It is during these times that your true mettle as an ex-smoker will be tested. When pushed to your limit, delay lighting a cigarette by 5 minutes and start another activity that you enjoy. According to the Riley Hospital for Children in Indiana, the urge to smoke will pass within 30 to 60 seconds whether you satisfy your craving with a cigarette or not. So, try with all your might to wait out the craving instead.

PRINCIPLE #169

Distract yourself with an alternative indulgence.

— ✳ —

Learn to extinguish the craving for a cigarette by substituting it with another indulgence. If eating a hot fudge sundae, taking yourself to the movies, or going on a shopping spree prevents you from lighting up, then so be it! It is important, however, that this sort of decadence should be reserved for only the most extreme circumstances—like when your entire cessation program is on the line. Acting on these impulses too often will create a different set of problems, such as eating too much or getting into credit-card debt. For the occasional blip in your program, though, distracting yourself with an indulgence can prevent you from falling back into your smoking habit.

PRINCIPLE #170

Never give up.

———————— ✳ ————————

It is important to recognize that by making the decision to quit smoking, you have become capable of realizing your goal. It may not happen right away, and you may stop and start smoking several times throughout your life, but the moment you made the decision to quit, you put yourself on the right path. Feel proud of that moment. Relive it often, and tell others about it. And, when faced with setbacks that cause you to doubt your purpose, think of the Buddhist Proverb that says, "If we are facing in the right direction, all we have to do is keep on walking." Indeed, no matter how many times it takes or how many relapses you must conquer, do not ever give up. Every day you do not smoke brings you closer to your goal of becoming a non-smoker for life.

REAPING THE BENEFITS OF A NON-SMOKING LIFESTYLE

The ancient Greek physician, Hippocrates, revolutionized medicine by viewing disease as the result of diet, lifestyle, and the environment instead of as punishment from God, as was the prevailing attitude of the time. Regarded as the "father of medicine," Hippocrates believed that illness was a by-product of imbalance in the body. As a result, he developed his treatments based on the concept of *physis*, meaning the belief that the body has the natural power to restore balance and heal itself.

Think of Hippocrates as you get used to your life as a non-smoker. When you smoked, your body's natural health was put off balance by the inhalation of noxious chemicals over a long period of time. However, by quitting, you allowed your body to flush toxins, restore its balance, and begin to heal. In addition to his faith in the body's natural ability to heal itself, Hippocrates also taught that one's living habits either exacerbated or diminished illness. To this end, he once said, "A wise man should consider that health is the greatest of human blessings, and learn how by his own thought to derive benefit from his illnesses." Indeed, as a recent ex-smoker you are blessed with having a new lease on life. Pausing to reflect on how your attitude affects the rate at which you restore your body's healthy balance is, in a sense, your Hippocratic duty.

As you will learn from the following simple principles, your body starts to recover from smoking immediately after your last cigarette. Within 2 days of quitting, your blood pressure returns to normal, nerve endings start to grow back, circulation improves, oxygen levels increase, heart rate slows, and your chance of having a heart attack is significantly reduced. If you stay quit, over time, your risk of developing heart disease and cancer will equal that of your non-smoking peers. With so many positive results it is no wonder that quitting is considered by every major health organization to be the best way to fix unhealthy imbalances caused by smoking.

Principle #171

Marvel at the first 24 hours of being a non-smoker.

---✳---

The first 24 hours after you quit smoking is a miraculous time. Incredibly, your body begins to heal within 20 minutes after your last cigarette! Your blood pressure will return to normal after 20 minutes, as will your pulse. After 8 hours, the concentration of carbon monoxide and nicotine levels in your blood are greatly decreased, the amount of oxygen in your blood returns to normal, and your risk for having a heart attack starts to fall. Ten hours after your last cigarette, carbon monoxide levels are halved and oxygen continues to reach your limbs and organs. After 24 hours, your ability to exercise improves. Put down that cigarette and let the healing begin!

Principle #172

Say goodbye to the smoker's hack.

— ✳ —

Within 2 weeks of quitting, your lungs begin to improve their functioning and breathing gets easier. Part of this process is the elimination of built-up toxins left by cigarette smoke. The leftover gunk must be cycled out of your lungs, but it can take awhile, depending on how much there is. According to Dr. Norman Edelman, a scientific advisor to the American Lung Association, "Within a few days to a week [after quitting], you start feeling better, and you start coughing up all that bad mucus you have down there." Exercise will hasten the "coming clean" process, but it will take a while for oxygen levels in your lungs to return to normal, so ease into an exercise program.

Principle #173

Come back to your senses.

———— ✳ ————

Just 48 hours after your last cigarette, your senses of taste and smell will be enhanced. As you put more distance between you and this habit, these senses will get even stronger. The world around you is likely to seem enhanced and brand-new. The scent of flowers, cologne, rain, and fresh-cut grass will overwhelm your senses. Food, too, will taste spicier, fresher, and have a zing that you will love. German philosopher Friedrich Nietzsche once wrote, "All credibility, all good conscience, all evidence of truth come only from the senses." Indeed, your senses are the gateway to the outside world and once you experience their revival, everything you smell, touch, and taste will be more enjoyable.

Principle #174

Enjoy your halved rate of having a heart attack.

---- ❈ ----

Quitting smoking is truly the best thing you can do for your heart. According to the Surgeon General's Health Report, after just 1 year of quitting smoking, the risk of developing smoking-related coronary heart disease is reduced by one-half. After 15 years, your risk of having a fatal heart attack is the same as those who have never smoked. This is because quitting smoking decreases the presence of fatty buildups in arteries, blood clots, coronary artery spasm, and heart rhythm problems, all caused by smoking. If you add a healthy diet, reduced stress, and exercise to your life, your chances of having a fatal heart attack will be even further reduced.

Principle #175

Take yourself off the list of people who are likely to suffer a stroke.

———————————— ✳ ————————————

Stroke is the third-leading cause of death in the U.S. A stroke is a type of cardiovascular disease that occurs when a blood vessel carrying oxygen to the brain bursts or is blocked by a blood clot. When blood is prevented from reaching the brain, that part of it is deprived of oxygen and begins to die. Strokes may result in paralysis, vision problems, memory loss, or even death. Since smoking causes blood clots, your risk of having a blood clot-related stroke once you quit is greatly reduced. In fact, the American Heart Association reports that within 5 to 15 years of quitting, an ex-smoker's risk of having a stroke is equal to that of non-smoker's.

PRINCIPLE #176

Relish in your decreased risk for developing lung cancer.

———————————— ❈ ————————————

A staggering 80 percent of lung cancer deaths in women and 90 percent in men are linked to smoking. In addition, there are more than 4,000 chemicals in the smoke of a single cigarette—60 of which are known carcinogens. And you do not just put yourself at risk by smoking—5 percent of new lung cancer diagnoses and about 3,000 lung cancer deaths are linked to secondhand smoke. As an ex-smoker, you have reduced the chances of both you and your non-smoking ones of developing lung cancers. Plus, if you quit before the age of 35, you reduce your risk for developing lung cancer by 90 percent, though quitting by the age of 50 also greatly reduces your risk.

Principle #177

Accept compliments on the improved look and feel of your hair and skin.

───────────── ✳ ─────────────

Smoking affects more than your health—it also changes your appearance by aging your skin as much as 20 years. The chemicals in cigarette smoke prevent red blood cells from getting oxygen around the body, which deprives your hair, skin, and nails of nutrients. This results in dry hair, yellowed nails, and premature wrinkles. Indeed, the hazards of smoking are most visible on the face. Studies show that smoking may cause collagen in the skin to break down making skin wrinkle and sag. One study found that smokers in their 40s had the same number of wrinkles as non-smokers in their 60s. As an ex-smoker, you will not only feel better, but look better too!

Principle #178

Make your belongings smoke-free, too!

❋

When you smoked, your clothes and belongings smoked with you. Tobacco smoke infiltrates every piece of fabric you own—clothes, towels, furniture, carpet, curtains, and car upholstery. In addition to the musty smell, smoke leaves a grimy residue on walls, windows, and other surfaces. As an ex-smoker, you'll want to be rid of this smell immediately! Try washing your walls and clothes in 1-gallon warm water, 1/2-cup plain ammonia, 1/4-cup white vinegar, and 1/4-cup washing soda. After you've cleaned your clothes and other fabrics you will smell fresh and clean for good! No more perfume showers after a cigarette! Once you quit smoking you are free to enter any situation with confidence.

Principle #179

Take the stairs again.

—— ✳ ——

Simple tasks such as walking up a flight of stairs were probably difficult for you when you smoked. Feeling out of breath after just a few steps likely sent you straight to the elevator. This pattern of breathlessness leading to avoidance of physical exertion significantly contributes to a smoker's deteriorating health. However, within just a few days of quitting smoking you are able to take the stairs—one step at a time. It may take a few weeks before you are able to do stairs without getting out of breath or coughing, but each time you take the stairs it will get easier. Track how you feel each time you use the stairs to measure the physical benefits of quitting smoking.

Principle #180

Make time for the things you love— you've got more of it than ever.

---- ❊ ----

The Smoking Cessation Health Center reports that each cigarette shaves 11 minutes from your lifespan. That means after just 1 week of smoking a pack a day, you have reduced the length of your life by 25 hours! However, the Centers for Disease Control and other organizations report that quitting smoking, eating a healthy diet rich in antioxidants, and exercising regularly not only stops this premature death clock, but may, in fact, reverse much of the damage. In addition to extending the length of your life, your ability to do more, play more, taste more, smell more, and feel better dramatically improves your quality of life.

Principle #181

Enjoy your freedom.

✳

Imagine waking up tomorrow and not needing a cigarette. Imagine after your morning coffee and stressful commute, eating a yogurt instead of stepping out to smoke. Imagine yourself stuck in a meeting for 3 hours and not sweating over when there will be a smoke break. Imagine flying cross-country and resting peacefully on the flight instead of pacing the aisle, dying for a cigarette. These scenarios are completely possible once you break your addiction to nicotine. Within 2 to 3 weeks of your last smoke, you will no longer be chained to a pack of cigarettes. No more obsessing over where your lighter is or how many cigarettes are left in the pack. From now on, your life is about freedom, spontaneity, and healthy choices that support your addiction-free lifestyle.

Principle #182

Love the extra money you've got.

※

According to Rutgers University, smokers blow so much of their money on cigarettes over the course of their life, a non-smoker's net worth is generally 50 percent more than light smokers, and double that of heavy smokers. However, pack-a-day smokers will increase their wealth by $1,820 annually after quitting—and be able to save nearly $20,000 in just 10 years! Even after you quit, continue to set aside money normally used to buy cigarettes. Open an account that allows your money to accrue interest, like a money-market account, IRA, or even just a regular savings account. Wherever you put this money, save it for retirement. Because you are going to live a longer, healthier life than you were as a smoker, you will need that money for the future!

Principle #183

Go on vacation again.

※

In a world that is increasingly non-smoking, quitting greatly enhances your travel experience. According to Consumer Affairs.com, the U.S., France, Ireland, Northern Ireland, Italy, Norway, Scotland, Sweden, Bhutan, Uganda, Finland, and Iceland are just a few countries that have public smoking bans in a significant number of cities. In addition, hotel chains like Marriott and Westin have gone smoke-free, as have most trains, taxis, and airplanes. When you were a smoker, the restrictions on smoking probably prevented you from taking a much-needed vacation. Now that you've quit, you have literally an entire world of travel possibilities. This is especially important for middle-aged men who increase their risk of heart attack by 30 percent when skipping vacation 5 years in a row.

PRINCIPLE #184

Know that your days of missing out are over.

───────── ❋ ─────────

How many interesting conversations have you missed because you went outside to smoke during a party? How often have you stood outside alone in the rain or in the dead of winter, all because you needed to take a smoke break? As an ex-smoker, your days of missing out are over. Never again will having a cigarette outside force you to miss the group photo or forgo the opportunity to hear the keynote address. You are now a member of the non-smoking community. Really notice how it feels to be fully invested in the activities going on around you. You are likely to be surprised at how much you truly missed out on when you were a smoker.

PRINCIPLE #185

Enjoy the feeling of self-pride.

— ✳ —

The minute you put out your last cigarette was when you began to experience that wonderful feeling of self-pride. Being proud of quitting smoking is one of its greatest benefits. People will want to hear your story, and will be impressed at your determination and hard work. You may even want to write about your experience for your local paper, or give a talk about what you've accomplished at your child's school, your workplace, or a local organization. At least once every day, remind yourself that you had the power to quit one of the most entrapping addictions known to man; that you took responsibility for your health and made the decision to live a long and vibrant life. Feels good, doesn't it?

STAYING SMOKE-FREE FOR LIFE

Inventor Alexander Graham Bell deeply valued the transformative power of self-actualization. Bell, who once said, "A man, as a general rule, owes very little to what he is born with—a man is what he makes himself," never gave up trying to create the telephone, even in the face of great adversity. Like Bell, in order to transform yourself into a non-smoker for life, you must live, breathe, and think like one, even under the most trying circumstances. In this way, you actualize your resolve to stay quit.

Your job up until now has been to wean yourself from cigarettes and make it through the initial days, weeks, and months as a non-smoker. After you conquer those challenges, your job becomes to stay smoke-free for life. Cultivating such a lifestyle will take work and may force you to make difficult decisions, such as limiting—or eliminating—time spent with people who tempt you to smoke. You should also steer clear of naysayers who will claim you are unable to stay smoke-free forever. In fact, quitting smoking may feel incredibly lonely at times. Dale Carnegie, author of *How to Win Friends and Influence People*, once wrote, "Most of the important things in the world have been accomplished by people who have kept on trying when there seemed to be no help at all." Indeed, you must constantly remind yourself that quitting smoking is one of the most important things in the world and one of the greatest things you have ever done.

This process requires the support of family and friends who believe in your ability to meet this lifelong challenge. Alexander Graham Bell, for example, was motivated by the encouragement of his friend, director of the Smithsonian Institution, Joseph Henry, who believed that Bell had, "the germ of a great invention." When Bell doubted his ability to continue with his experiments, Henry simply told him to "Get it!" Finding the "Joseph Henry" who will nudge you forward when you feel like slipping back is one of many ways to keep you from smoking. For more useful tips on how to stay smoke-free for life, incorporate the following principles into your cessation-maintenance program.

Principle #186

Never forget how hard it was to quit.

———————————— ❉ ————————————

Quitting smoking may be the most difficult challenge you have ever come up against. The hell endured during the weeks of withdrawal is something most smokers would not wish on their worst enemy—sleepless nights, headaches, irritability, nausea, anxiety, and battling the constant urge to smoke. Remember this time. Meditate on it occasionally and try to re-experience it on a visceral level. Remind yourself that you do not ever want to be in that position again. As French author André Gide once wrote, "In hell there is no other punishment than to begin over and over again the tasks left unfinished in your lifetime." In this spirit, remind yourself of how hard it was to quit.

Principle #187

Stay conscious of your reasons for quitting.

✳

One ex-smoker remembers how, a decade ago, she asked her son what he wanted for Christmas. He asked her to quit smoking and, as a result, she hasn't touched a cigarette in 10 years. Like this parent, the reason you initially wanted to quit was likely a powerful one. Keep it close to your heart and mind as you move through life as a non-smoker. If you quit because you had a heart-attack scare, never let the fear you felt become dull. If you quit because you were constantly ostracized for your habit, never let the memory of standing alone outside of work or a party leave you. Staying conscious of your reason for first quitting will keep you quit for life.

PRINCIPLE #188

Volunteer to help someone else quit smoking.

———————————— ✳ ————————————

As you think back over your quitting experience, remember the people who supported you through difficult times as well as those who celebrated the minutes, hours, and days you went without smoking. Take what you learned from them and pay that supportive knowledge forward. Helping someone else quit smoking not only helps them but forcefully reminds you how difficult quitting actually is. As one study in *Law and Contemporary Problems* found, "Volunteers [have] a lower mortality hazard than non-volunteers," because their work reminds them of the reality of addiction.

PRINCIPLE #189

Have regular health evaluations.

———————————— ❖ ————————————

Giving up cigarettes is one part of an overall commitment to a healthier lifestyle. One way to evaluate the effects on your health is to see your doctor at least once a year for an annual physical. As an ex-smoker, you may need to see your doctor more than this to monitor your cardiovascular and respiratory health. Keeping tabs on coughs, palpitations, and other symptoms that do not go away is important, not to mention an excellent smoking deterrent. Each time you visit your doctor, let it reaffirm your decision to quit by noting the improvements to your blood pressure, pulse, cholesterol, and lung capacity. Plus, your doctor will likely tell you over and over that quitting smoking was the best thing you ever could have done for your health!

Principle #190

Celebrate milestones and anniversaries.

After everything you have gone through to quit smoking, you deserve to celebrate! In fact, rewarding milestones and celebrating anniversaries is an integral part of your lifelong non-smoking-maintenance program. When you commemorate important dates, you acknowledge your hard work and track the increasing distance between you and smoking. Some suggestions for how to acknowledge your achievements are to quietly reflect after the first 6 months; have a party 1 year from your quit date; donate to a cancer charity on each anniversary of your quit date; participate in a walk for your favorite cause; and take a trip every 5 years that you remain smoke-free.

Principle #191

Train for a physical challenge.

———————————— ✳ ————————————

Stay smoke-free by making it a point to train for some sort of physical endeavor, like a triathlon or a backpacking trip. This is another way to mark the huge gains you have made since you last smoked. When you first quit smoking, it was probably difficult for you to walk up a flight of stairs without getting winded. If engage in challenging training programs, you will amaze yourself and others with how much you are able to accomplish. Do 20 minutes of cardio daily, try kayaking, take surf lessons, train for a half-marathon, hike the peak of a local mountain, bike to work, take scuba lessons, or learn to ski. These physical challenges will keep you fit and keep you too busy to even think about smoking!

Principle #192

Remember to think of yourself as a "recovering smoker."

———————————— ✳ ————————————

The kiss of death for any ex-smoker is thinking that they have completed their smoking-cessation program. In reality, an ex-smoker's work is never done. Like with alcohol, drug, and food addictions, giving up smoking requires lifelong maintenance. While it will get increasingly easier to stay smoke-free, never think of yourself as being completely out of the woods with regards to your nicotine addiction. Remember that tobacco companies want you to smoke again—so much so that they spend billions on advertising to lure you back. Remain humbled by your addiction and committed to your program, and you will succeed in staying smoke-free for life.

Principle #193

Feel alive, rather than deprived.

---- ❋ ----

Staying smoke-free for life requires you to avoid feeling frustrated, tempted, resentful, or deprived of cigarettes. To get to this place, remind yourself that you chose to quit smoking in order to live a better, longer life. So live it! Continue to support your choice to become a non-smoker by making decisions that are consistent with your new, capable persona—such as learning new skills, challenging yourself, and growing. Use the determination you showed during quitting smoking to other ends in your life. Let your newfound strength inspire you to change careers, start a relationship, or travel around the world. Each cigarette sucked 11 minutes from your life, so vow to make the most of every extra 11 minutes you earn as a non-smoker.

Principle #194

Maintain a healthy lifestyle.

——————— ✳ ———————

It makes sense that maintaining a healthy lifestyle discourages smoking. In fact, surveys show that vegetarians who regularly practice yoga and meditation have the lowest rates of nicotine addiction out of all Americans. It seems as though the work of shopping, prepping, and cooking fresh, nutritious food, combined with the discipline and well-being established in yoga is incompatible with tobacco use. You don't have to become a vegetarian or a yogi to keep yourself smoke-free for life, however. Avoiding junk and fast-food; limiting sweets, caffeine, and alcohol; doing some form of daily exercise; and practicing stress-management skills can be enough to make your permanent answer "no" when offered a cigarette.

Principle #195

End your preoccupation with smoking.

— ✳ —

Smoking-cessation expert Charles F. Wetherall advises ex-smokers, "When we stop thinking about not smoking, it becomes a lot easier not to smoke." It is true there will come a time when you make it through an entire day without once thinking about smoking (or not smoking). Indeed, your life as a non-smoker will come naturally after working to fill your life with activities that are both satisfying and good for you. However, it will take effort and time—possibly years—before you are able to pass your days without the thought of cigarettes. Be patient, work hard, and keep busy and you will get to the point where you participate in activities because you genuinely enjoy them, not just because they distract you from smoking.

Principle #196

Hug and kiss often.

※

Stay smoke free by hugging and kissing you family and friends every chance you get. The benefits of frequent expressions of affection are plentiful. Expressing your feelings to your loved ones makes them feel safe and appreciated. It limits regrets, allows you to show off your fresh breath and clean smell, and increases your chances of staying quit by minimizing depression and stress. Professor Kory Floyd of Arizona State University's Hugh Downs School of Human Communication has said, "Highly affectionate people tend to have better mental health and less stress. They also react to stress better." Floyd would agree with every smoking-cessation expert that stress management and psychological well-being are crucial to the ex-smoker's continued success.

PRINCIPLE #197

Realize that being smoke-free helps you climb life's ladder.

———————— ✴ ————————

In addition to saving the money spent on cigarettes, staying smoke-free for life can actually help you earn a higher salary. In fact, studies show that non-smokers are thought of as more desirable candidates for higher-paying jobs. A survey conducted by the Society for Human Resource Management found that a statistically significant percentage of employers prefer hiring non-smokers, and a few employers will not hire smokers at all. Some companies even ask smokers to contribute more money to their health insurance than non-smokers. The next time you are looking for a higher-paying job, be proud to list "non-smoker" on your application.

Principle #198

Frame your quit contract and have someone you love bear witness.

Earlier in this book, you made a quit contract with yourself. After you have made it through the unstable valley of quitting and on to surer footing, make permanent the code you signed. Buy a beautiful frame for your contract and hang it the way you would a diploma, Ketubah, or other important certificate. Ask a loved one—a friend, spouse, or child—to observe this framing and hanging ceremony. This makes your pledge public as well as personal. Make sure to hang your quit contract somewhere visible where visitors to your home will see it and ask you about it. The more people you tell your inspiring story to, the better.

Principle #199

Do not envy social smokers.

❊

At one time or another, many ex-smokers have lamented, "I wish I could just smoke socially like so-and-so does." But as French author François Duc de La Rochefoucauld wrote, "Our envy always lasts longer than the happiness of those we envy." This is especially true of smoking. The actual satisfaction of the social smoker's habit lasts only 3 to 5 minutes, yet an ex-smoker will ponder the perceived enjoyment for days! Looking fondly upon smoking of any kind is detrimental to your ability to stay tobacco-free. Instead, be motivated to remain a non-smoker by remembering that *you* are the lucky one who broke free from nicotine addiction—and from all of the consequences that go along with a smoking habit of any kind.

Principle #200

Learn your Achilles' heel and respect it.

—— ✳ ——

An Achilles' heel—named after the mythological Greek character Achilles, who was invincible save for one spot on his heel—is a fatal weakness in spite of overall strength. Staying smoke-free for life requires you to identify what your Achilles' heel is, and stay away from it. For some people, their Achilles' heel might be hanging out with their old smoking friends. For others, it might be a particular brand of alcohol. Still others might feel prone to smoking when they hear a particular song or visit a certain part of town. In such situations, your guard is likely to crumble. Keep yourself in one invincible piece by identifying your supreme weakness and avoiding it altogether.

Additional
Information and Ideas

The following pages contain exercises, tips, and information that will help you to quit smoking for good. Use these materials to support your cessation program. The exercises here will help you to get a handle on your smoking habit, make a plan to quit, and monitor your progress after Quit Day.

The following pages will improve your chances of giving up cigarettes by empowering you to take action over your addiction. They also provide ready-made tools, such as a quit contract, which you can use to put your commitment to quit down on paper. Furthermore, valuable information on nicotine replacement (NRT) products is provided to help you understand your options and choose the best NRT for your individual needs.

Tracking Your Smoking Habits
This exercise helps you identify the various components that make up your smoking habit. Learning why and when you smoke is necessary for creating a successful quit plan.

Ten Activities to Substitute for a Cigarette
Knowing what to put in your hand instead of a cigarette is critical for avoiding slipups and relapses.

Drafting a Quit Contract
This exercise helps you draft that critical quit contract, the document that firms up your commitment to quit smoking. Treat it as legally binding and have a loved one bear witness for additional accountability.

Nicotine Replacement Therapy (NRT)
Studies show that use of NRT in combination with other sources of support more than doubles a smoker's chances of quitting for good. This exercise familiarizes you with various NRT options.

Keeping Track of Your Progress

Document your journey to becoming a non-smoker in a blank journal. Acknowledge every good decision, educational mistake, and valuable milestone as you get further and further from your last cigarette. These pages will give you some starting points for keeping this important journal. Brainstorm your own questions and record any thoughts, hopes, or worries you might have. Be proud of your journey!

Tracking Your Smoking Habits

Before you make a quit plan, you must get a handle on your smoking habit. Doing so gives you a comprehensive, subjective view of your habit, allowing you to figure out the best angle from which to attack it. The best way to form an attack plan is to track your behavior and habit over the course of a week.

Get a piece of paper and create a chart with space for 7 days of the week. For each day, write down the times when you smoke—include the first and last cigarettes of the day and every one in between. Log your mood while smoking: were you angry, sad, nervous, excited, or anxious? Next, keep track of what you ate and drank just before smoking. Note who you smoked with and what you were doing while you had a cigarette. Were you talking, walking, sitting, standing, driving, pacing, or doing some other activity with your hands? Write down where you smoked—at work, in the car, walking to the store, at a bar, etc. Finally, at the end of each day, write down how many cigarettes are left in your pack.

Keeping accurate records of your daily smoking habit will reveal patterns of behavior that will help you to shape a quit plan. For example, you will likely note that you smoke at the same time every day, with the same people, in the same places. This gives you an idea of where you must focus your efforts to create alternatives to the usual temptations you face every day that encourage you to smoke.

Ten Activities to Substitute for a Cigarette

Two things that all smoking-cessation programs agree upon are the concepts of "delay and distract" when trying to quit smoking. Especially in the first few weeks, when withdrawal symptoms are gnawing at you to smoke, using the delay and distract tactic may be the only way to prevent you from giving in to temptation.

Delaying having a cigarette buys you time before lighting up. It is a simple yet effective technique, because the longer you are able to go between cigarettes, you decrease your addiction to nicotine. By distracting yourself from the urge to smoke you occupy your mind until the craving passes, addressing your mental or emotional attachment to smoking.

Use the following list of substitutions whenever you are tempted to smoke. You should also come up with your own list to add variety and help you remain smoke-free.

1. Clean!

Scour the bathroom, scrub the kitchen floor, vacuum the house, clean your windows, or wash the car. These activities take time and exert physical energy. By the time you are finished, your craving will have passed and you will have the satisfaction of a clean house and car.

2. Organize your environment.

This can be done at home or at work. Shred old mail, organize files, rearrange furniture, move your computer, empty your desk, organize closets, make donation piles, alphabetize CDs or DVDs, put photos in albums, rewrite your address book, or make a file with which to track expenses. Projects are a great way to lose yourself and forget about your craving. Make sure they are satisfying and require at least 10 to 15 minutes of your time for completion.

3. Exercise.

Go for a walk, jog, or run. Do 20 minutes of cardio, such as kickboxing, aerobics, rollerblading, jumping rope, swimming, rowing, or dancing. Do 3 reps of 12 bicep curls with weights. Do as many pushups as you are able. Get down and do 25 sit-ups. Exercising not only occupies your mind and body but will help keep your weight down and improve your overall health.

4. **Enjoy a healthy snack.**
Always have crunchy snacks on hand, such as carrots, celery, jicama, almonds, walnuts, bagel chips, and apples. In addition, keep foods on hand that have been statistically proven to keep you from smoking, such as oranges, yogurt, low-fat string cheese, raisins, licorice, bananas, and grapes. Healthy snacking helps deal with the oral fixation of smoking and gives you something to do with your hands. By making smart choices, you will keep your weight in check and avoid foods that tempt you to smoke.

5. **Talk to someone you love.**
Call a friend or family member when you are tempted to smoke. Sometimes, expressing the desire to smoke out loud to a trusted friend is enough to get through the period of temptation.

6. Keep a journal.

Writing through a craving is an excellent way to identify why you want to smoke. Pay special attention to physical cravings versus emotional and mental ones. Keep track of your mood, the foods you ate, and whether you drank caffeinated or alcoholic beverages. Revisit each entry later to make connections and identify areas that still need work.

7. Go to the movies.

When temptation strikes, get yourself to a place where you will be busy, distracted, and unable to smoke, even if you tried. Examples include movie theaters, churches, government buildings, museums, hospitals, animal shelters, nursing homes, aquariums, and shopping malls.

8. Scream!

When you are tempted to smoke, you may just feel like screaming. So, go for it! Scream your head off while driving, or blast the radio and yell the lyrics to your favorite song. Go into a vacant office at work and yell your head off. Let your family know you'll be in the bathroom, turn on all the faucets and shout until the craving has passed. Expressing pent-up energy in this way is both cathartic and healthy and will definitely purge your craving to smoke.

9. **Meditate.**
Practicing relaxation through meditation is a proven method of becoming centered and calm. Taking time out of your day to meditate and get grounded in your new life as a non-smoker will give you the presence of mind to deal with cravings as they arise. You can also use "walking meditation" to focus on your breath and the number of steps taken until the craving passes.

10. **Allow for a different indulgence.**
There are times when your urge to smoke will be so great that the only way to avoid giving in is to do something really indulgent. Though this method should be reserved for extreme cases, once in a while it is necessary to eat a hot fudge sundae or go shopping for something you have wanted to buy. If you do this too often, however, you simply replace smoking with other bad habits. So, use this tip sparingly!

Drafting a Quit Contract

Make your commitment to quit official! Create a quit contract similar to the one on the following page, or modify the language to suit your own goals and situation. Have someone you care about sign as your witness. Being held accountable to you, the contract, and your witness will greatly increase your chances of success. When you have been quit long enough to count yourself as a true ex-smoker (usually after 6 months or a year), frame this document and hang it on the wall of your home.

My Quit-Smoking Contract

I _____ , commit to giving up
cigarettes. I realize this will be difficult, but I am up to the challenge.
I recognize and understand the diseases I have put myself at risk for,
and I am ready to stop risking and start healing. I understand that
my family and friends are here to support me, but that ultimately it
is up to me to quit and stay quit.

- I vow to ask for help when I need it.
- I promise to try my hardest to avoid temptation.
- I vow to seek any and all alternatives to smoking.
- I promise to eat healthily and avoid foods that tempt me
  to smoke.
- I commit myself to a long and healthy life.
- I acknowledge that by signing this contract I also make
  these promises to my witness.

_____   _____
Signature   Date

_____   _____
Witness   Date

Nicotine Replacement Therapy

Nicotine replacement therapy (NRT) has been shown to double the chances of successfully quitting smoking when used properly and with other methods of support, such as cessation programs, quit groups, online chat rooms, family and friends, and quit buddies. Indeed, it is the official position of the American Heart Association that "nicotine transdermal patches and other nicotine substitution drug products, such as nicotine gum, can help smokers quit when used as part of a comprehensive smoking-cessation program."

The following section will provide more information on available NRTs. Note that some of these products require a prescription, and users should be monitored by their doctor throughout the length of treatment. In addition, keep in mind that use of NRT is a temporary means for reducing your addiction to nicotine over time and that your ultimate goal is to be completely free of nicotine addiction.

- **Nicotine Patch.** Available over the counter (OTC) and by prescription. Nicotine is released in a constant flow from an adhesive patch you stick on your body and wear for 24 hours. The patch slows absorption of nicotine into the blood as it can take up to 3 hours to pass through all the skin layers. Potential side effects include skin irritation, dizziness, nausea, headaches, and increased heart rate.

- **Nicotine Gum.** OTC. Nicotine is absorbed by chewing gum. It reaches the brain faster than the patch, but slower than smoking. The gum is to be chewed and "parked" between your teeth and cheeks for maximum absorption. If you continuously chew the gum, you will swallow the nicotine and decrease its effectiveness. You must not eat or drink within 15 minutes before and after chewing the gum. Usual dosing is 10 to 15 pieces a day, but never chew more than 30 in a 24-hour period. Side effects may include stomach aches, dental problems, nausea, and headaches.

- **Nicotine Lozenge.** OTC. Nicotine is released over a period of 30 minutes by sucking on a hard candy. Chewing the lozenge releases all of the nicotine at once and may cause upset stomach and other adverse side effects. Dosing should not exceed more than 20 lozenges in a 24-hour period and the user should cease using lozenges after 12 weeks. Like nicotine gum, do not eat or drink within 15 minutes before or after sucking on a lozenge. Side effects may include sore gums, teeth, and throat, and upset stomach.

- **Nicotine Nasal Spray.** By prescription only. Nicotine is rapidly absorbed into the brain through a nasal spray. User should not exceed 40 doses per day. Side effects may include sore nose and throat.

- **Nicotine Inhaler.** By prescription only. The inhaler is puffed like a cigarette and releases nicotine into the mouth. Nicotine is more slowly absorbed than by smoking, but faster than other NRTs. It is recommended that the user continuously puffs on the inhaler for 20 minutes to receive maximum benefits. Treatment lasts 12 weeks, but no more than 16. Side effects may include sore throat and mouth, and coughing.

- **Non-nicotine Pills.**
  - » By prescription only. Bupropion hydrochloride (Zyban or Wellbutrin). Treatment is begun a week from your quit date and continues for between 7 and 12 weeks. If you do not experience relief by week 7, treatment is discontinued. Side effects may include dizziness, insomnia, and dry mouth.

  - » By prescription only. Varenicline tartrate (Chantix). Treatment lasts for 12 weeks and works by reducing the pleasure of smoking as well as the intensity of withdrawal symptoms. Treatment may be extended to another 12 weeks to increase success. Side effects may include nausea, headache, vomiting, gas, insomnia, unusual dreams, and noticeable differences in your sense of taste.

KEEPING TRACK OF YOUR PROGRESS

Purchase a blank journal so that you may track your progress and note your successes over a period of 6 months. This journal will help you feel confident in your ability to remain smoke-free and will give you a motivator to look back on throughout your journey.

The following are examples of things you will want to record in your journal:

- Keep track of every time you wanted to smoke, but didn't
- Note the money you've saved as a result of quitting
- Write down your smoking triggers to then avoid them
- Write down a positive affirmation that will encourage you to stay quit. An example is, "I know that I have the power to stay quit, because it has already been 35 days since my last cigarette!"
- Record minor setbacks and how you were able to deal with them
- Note the special people who have supported you
- Brainstorm hands-on activities you might try
- Record your accomplishments and milestones

CONCLUSION

Hopefully, the journey that *Simple Principles® to Quit Smoking* has taken you on has caused you to realize that quitting smoking, though difficult, is entirely possible. You should also understand that it took years to build up your habit, and defeating your nicotine addiction will be a process that takes time and planning. However, with this book at your disposal, you eliminate much of the guesswork involved in creating your personalized smoking-cessation plan.

Moreover, you should feel hopeful about your prospects of giving up smoking for good, because this book has shown you that you can take the reins from your habit and stop letting it control you. By deconstructing the components that comprise your habit you have learned how to deal with them on an individual basis. You have also learned how to use visualization to cull the best images of what being a non-smoker looks and feels like. In addition, you now understand that prior to giving up smoking you must believe you will succeed. And finally, you have learned the serious health risks of continuing to smoke, as well as the many and immediate benefits of quitting.

The hundreds of reasons for quitting contained within these pages have hopefully encouraged you to develop the willpower to resist temptation. Indeed, learning there are steps you can take to build up to quitting, such as creating a plan and tapering off, should significantly reduce your fears and prepare you to cope without cigarettes. The tips, tricks, and ideas contained within *Simple Principles® to Quit Smoking* have set you up for the best possible outcome. Follow the 200-plus pieces of advice to quit smoking and stay nicotine-free for life!

TELL US YOUR STORY

Simple Principles® to Quit Smoking has changed the lives of countless people, helping them quit smoking and stay smoke-free better than they ever imagined. Now we want to hear your story about how this book has helped you in your quest to stop smoking.

Tell us ...
• Why did you purchase this book?
• Had you tried to quit smoking unsuccessfully before?
• How did this book help you quit successfully?
• How did this book change your life?
• Which principles did you like the most?
• What did you like most about this book?
• Would you recommend this book to others?

Email us your response at info@wspublishinggroup.com or write to us at:

WS Publishing Group
7290 Navajo Road, Suite 207
San Diego, CA 92119

Please include your name and an email address and/or phone number where you can be reached.

Please let us know if WS Publishing may or may not use your story and/or name in future book titles, and if you would be interested in participating in radio or TV interviews.

Great Titles in the
SIMPLE PRINCIPLES™ SERIES

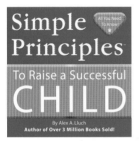

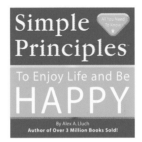

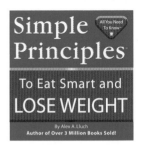

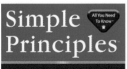

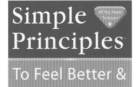

More Great Titles in the
SIMPLE PRINCIPLES™ SERIES

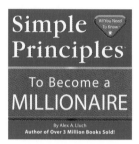

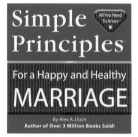

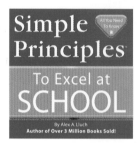

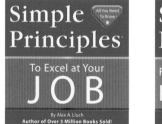

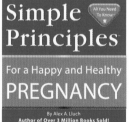

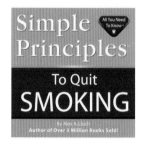

LOG ON TO **WSPublishingGroup.com** TO CHECK FOR
RELEASE DATES ON THESE AND FUTURE TITLES.

Other Best-Selling Books
by Alex A. Lluch

HOME & FINANCE

- The Very Best Home Improvement Guide & Document Organizer
- The Very Best Home Buying Guide & Document Organizer
- The Very Best Home Selling Guide & Document Organizer
- The Very Best Budget & Finance Guide with Document Organizer
- The Ultimate Home Journal & Organizer
- The Ultimate Home Buying Guide & Organizer

BABY JOURNALS & PARENTING

- The Complete Baby Journal Organizer & Keepsake
- Keepsake of Love Baby Journal
- Snuggle Bears Baby Journal Keepsake & Organizer
- Humble Bumbles Baby Journal
- Simple Principles to Raise a Successful Child

CHILDREN'S BOOKS

- I Like to Learn: Alphabet, Numbers, Colors & Opposites
- Alexander, It's Time for Bed!
- Do I Look Good in Color?
- Zoo Clues Animal Alphabet
- Animal Alphabet: Slide & Seek the ABC's
- Counting Chameleon
- Big Bugs, Small Bugs

LOG ON TO **WSPublishingGroup.com** TO CHECK FOR
RELEASE DATES ON THESE AND FUTURE TITLES.

More Best-Selling Books
by Alex A. Lluch

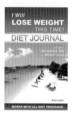

COOKING, FITNESS & DIET

- The Very Best Cooking Guide & Recipe Organizer
- Easy Cooking Guide & Recipe Organizer
- Get Fit Now! Workout Journal
- Lose Weight Now! Diet Journal & Organizer
- I Will Lose Weight This Time! Diet Journal
- The Ultimate Pocket Diet Journal

WEDDING PLANNING

- The Ultimate Wedding Planning Kit
- The Complete Wedding Planner & Organizer
- Easy Wedding Planner, Organizer & Keepsake
- Easy Wedding Planning Plus
- Easy Wedding Planning
- The Ultimate Wedding Workbook & Organizer
- The Ultimate Wedding Planner & Organizer
- Making Your Wedding Beautiful, Memorable & Unique
- Planning the Most Memorable Wedding on Any Budget
- My Wedding Journal, Organizer & Keepsake
- The Ultimate Wedding Planning Guide
- The Ultimate Guide to Wedding Music
- Wedding Party Responsibility Cards

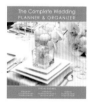

LOG ON TO **WSPUBLISHINGGROUP.COM** TO CHECK FOR RELEASE DATES ON THESE AND FUTURE TITLES.